KID JENSEN
FOR THE RECORD

DAVID JENSEN

FOREWORD BY
PAUL GAMBACCINI

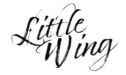

ISBN 978-1-911273-95-0

Published by Little Wing

An imprint of
Mango Books
18 Soho Square
London W1D 3QL

www.LittleWingBooks.com

KID JENSEN

FOR THE RECORD

To my grandchildren.

CONTENTS

ACKNOWLEDGEMENTS

Thanks to David Lloyd for his patience and hard work in helping me bring this project to fruition, and to Adam Wood at Little Wing Books for his enthusiasm.

My gratitude too to Alan Bailey, Paul Burnett, Trevor Dann, Golly Gallagher, Peter Monnery, Nathan Morley, Parkinson's UK, and Frank Rodgers, who helped check my stories and jog my memory.

Last but not least, my thanks to my family and friends for their love and support.

TRIBUTES

You can't bluff on live radio so, as a listener, I always thought David Jensen would be a nice man! But then, when I found myself living close to him, our kids all growing up together and working alongside him for years, I realised he was so much more than that. His love of radio is huge, his knowledge of music enormous, but above all he is a genuine, kind decent man. In a tough media world, he is one of the good guys. CHRIS TARRANT

○

Kid has both credibility and likeability in spades. A really clever but funny guy, he is hugely respected by the artists and loved by his colleagues. I have so much affection for Kid, and it's great to document his fascinating life. PAUL BURNETT

○

I have always admired David Jensen's talent and professionalism, but I've also had the pleasure of knowing him as a friend for more than three decades. He was so encouraging and helpful to me early in my career – something I'll never forget – and is simply is one of the nicest people you will ever meet; warm-hearted, good-humoured and, above all, a very kind person. It's a rare thing to find a person that everybody likes and respects – David is that man. PAUL McKENNA

○

I am so proud to have David as a true friend, plus I have so much admiration for his achievements in both his career and his life. With a radio voice that is the envy of presenters everywhere plus youthful looks that surpass even that of Cliff Richard, coupled with that of a vast knowledge of both music and sport, David 'Kid' Jensen is also an extremely kind and caring man in every respect. Which makes me wonder… just how annoyingly perfect can one human being possibly be! RICK WAKEMAN

○

Our first album *Wishbone Ash* was released in 1970 and some chap called Kid Jensen at Radio Luxembourg was playing it, big time. He did the same in 1971 with our second album *Pilgrimage*, and yet again in 1972 when *Argus* was released. Around this period we travelled out to Luxembourg to do a live recording at the radio station and met Kid in person, giving us the chance to say "thanks" for the wonderful exposure we had received from his Rock Chart. We lost contact for many decades, but then one day my son Tom arrived home and asked me if I knew a disc jockey by the name of 'Kid' – I was delighted to hear that my son was good mates with Viktor, Kid and Gudrun's lad, and that they played in the same football team. I had the pleasure of rolling up at their next match, strolling down the line to where Kid was standing, and saying "Fancy bumping into you here, Kid!" It was indeed a pleasure to see this great man again. I use the word 'great', because as the Sixties gave way to the Seventies music coverage on radio and TV was a bit sad and way behind. It took a man with vision to give the music on radio a good kick up the backside. In that respect he is up there with Alan Freeman, John Peel, Jo Whiley and I'm sure a good few others. For me, being a creative musician, I hold them all in high regard. They all deserve medals. MARTIN TURNER, WISHBONE ASH

o

Growing up he was an icon, with that effervescence and that voice. When I arrived at Palace years ago he was easily the most famous person I knew, and I never imagined we'd end up being friends. He was so supportive. I have a genuine love for the guy. IAN WRIGHT

o

David is easy to like, with his warmth, his soothing voice and calm manner. His glass is always half-full, and he tackled most obstacles placed in his way on the way up as a DJ, just like he is now tackling Parkinson's. He's a person who can make anyone feel at ease, and I'm proud to call him my friend. With the industry he's been in, and the people he's met, this book will be a must-read for music and football fans alike. David, you've interviewed many a star, but in reality, *you* really are the star. MARK BRIGHT

o

My connection to Parkinson's UK was originally through my brother-in-law, and I've been honoured to have worked with this wonderful charity since he was first diagnosed. One of the great pleasures it has brought me has been meeting some extraordinary and genuinely inspiring people, and the charismatic, clever and relentlessly delightful David Jensen has to be one of the best. Inevitably, in my position I come across many differing reactions to a diagnosis of Parkinson's, and I'm always amazed when that reaction, as with David, is to help, unselfishly, the Parkinson's community. I am privileged to be able to work with him to improve the lot of all those whom we support. JANE ASHER, PRESIDENT OF PARKINSON'S UK

FOREWORD

BY PAUL GAMBACCINI

I first met Kid Jensen in late 1972 when I was writing an article for *Rolling Stone* about radio in the UK. I sat in on Kid's late-night show, after which he took me to a local disco. A record came on, and he said 'I've interviewed this singer. He is going to be a star, and this record is going to be a hit.' He was right on both counts. The song was 'Whiskey in the Jar' by Thin Lizzy. The lead singer was Phil Lynott.

I thus had an early indication of Kid's talent-scouting ability. But I could have no idea that within a few years we would be back-to-back on Radio 1, on either side of noon. As fellow North Americans, Kid from Canada and yours truly from the United States, we were often referred to in the same breath and shared our first Radio 1 calendar page, which in the mid-Seventies was a big deal.

Neither of us could believe our luck, having travelled from thousands of miles away to be broadcasting to the entire United Kingdom and other nations in signal range. We called ourselves the Paranoia Twins, looking over our shoulders to see if any Radio 1 newcomers were sneaking up on us, ready to take our time slots.

Kid Jensen has honoured us all with his best tasteful work. Not only did I have the privilege of deputising for him on both Radio 1 and Capital Radio, I had a turn at presenting a network album chart show on commercial radio that was a follow-on from his successful Network Chart Show.

No matter the twists and turns of our broadcasting careers, management could never keep the Paranoia Twins apart. Our friendship continues to this day. I can't think of a better friend to be paranoid with.

PREFACE

On-air, I have never been a radio presenter to talk about my own life too much, but now, facing the challenges of Parkinson's, it seemed like an appropriate time to tell my story whilst I can. It's a privileged one, dominated by good luck, good friends and happiness.

The power of radio is clear, and it has been my privilege to play a part. From the origins of the DJ in the dance halls to the role that presenters have played on-air in more recent times, it is humbling to know that, for so many people, we have been the soundtrack to their lives, and our voices and the tracks we played are as much a part of their own stories as the places they went and the people they knew.

A London cab driver was the catalyst for eventually rushing into print. As we paused at the traffic lights on a journey to Waterloo station, he swung his head around and reminded me of some of the people I had encountered in my life, and suggested I must write down the tales. Flattered by his show of enthusiasm but rather wishing he would focus on the road ahead, he then reminded me that the people who would most value my account are getting no younger, and that I should hurry.

I have.

DOES THIS HURT?

Ambling down the road near my home on a sunny Surrey day, I noticed a family approaching me from the other direction. A mother with her two children, and a beautiful long-haired Dachshund trailing behind.

I smiled as our paths crossed, and looked down fondly at their furry friend.

'That's a really lovely dog,' I said.

'What dog?' she replied.

Hallucinations are a side-effect of the drugs I must take for my Parkinson's. The medication helps to manage the symptoms of this incurable condition.

As a kid, I had always been a lazy walker and my mother nagged me not to drag my feet. The trait became more pronounced as I grew older and, in recent years, I started to shake as I stretched in the morning on waking. It became one of those puzzles you plan to mention to a doctor – one day.

It was a rigorous Royal Marine, rather than my doctor, who prompted me to take the symptoms more seriously. Embarking on a fitness drive whilst working for Smooth Radio in Salford, I bravely signed up for some PE courses the Forces were running, which demanded a cursory medical assessment before the torture began. The muscular Marine moved my hand around. 'Does this hurt?' 'No,' I replied. He moved it again. Still no pain. He tried another arm wrench, but despite his determination to make me wince, I felt nothing. In the tone of voice you do not ignore, he then cautioned that there was a medical issue and recommended I get it checked out.

Noel Gallagher was leaving the Harley Street surgery just as I entered. We nodded on the steps. A bizarre coincidence rather than a premature hallucination.

Inside, a neurologist questioned me carefully before shuffling his papers and failing to look into my eyes as he delivered his blunt yet accurate verdict. I was to consult a second neurologist too; not because I wanted verification, I simply found the bedside manner of the first off-putting for this most sensitive of conversations.

The team in white jackets prodded and probed and subjected me to a kaleidoscope of tests. The MRI scan suggested all was well; then came the SPECT scan providing 3D images of my insides.

The doctor studied the results. 'That's fine,' he said, pointing his pencil at one unrecognisable blob. 'And that's good too,' he said, pointing at another. 'Ah,' he exclaimed, pointing somewhere else, just near the top of my head.

Parkinson's was diagnosed. 'It could be worse,' he reassured. 'Now we are going on a journey together.' I gather that has become a curious medical cliché for such situations, trying to make the worst day of your life sound like a jolly package holiday. No tests can show conclusively that you have Parkinson's. Doctors base a diagnosis on your symptoms, medical history and a detailed physical examination.

None of us knows for sure whether the anticipated path for the remainder of our life will be as expected. It could change tomorrow for any one of us. And we wonder whether we would be able to cope – and how.

I was scared.

I was devastated.

I was angry.

And, yes, you ask yourself selfishly: 'Why me?'

Google learnt exactly what was on my mind as the news began to sink in over the first weeks. I had wrongly thought Parkinson's to be a disease for old people, and the start of a long slope to the pearly gates. Reading all I could about my condition, I drew little comfort from learning I was unlikely to die from Parkinson's itself, but from the symptoms, such as not being able to swallow food, or falling dangerously, or something equally cheery. I would recommend closing the browser and talking things through with a doctor instead.

The experts advised me to tell no-one of my condition: 'Don't tell your wife, your family, your best friend. Nobody.' They suggested that people would persist in asking 'How are you?' over what would be a lengthy journey. The proposed silence seemed an odd strategy to someone like me. I quite like people in Waitrose asking how I am.

Regardless, the news was shared with my wife Guðrún and a close doctor friend in hushed voices, before five years of subterfuge, guilt and loneliness began. Even aside from the doctor's advice, I feared that others might think less of me were they to be aware of my situation. My shaking hands were secreted quickly in my pockets when I began a conversation, and I found excuses to explain the many pill bottles I fiddled with in the studio every few hours. I shall forever be grateful to the small group of people with whom I did share my news, in confidence, for keeping knowledge of my condition to themselves, and allowing me to choose the time and place to say more.

Talking to younger members of the family demanded a deep breath, and a book called *My Grandad Has Parkinson's* proved as useful as it sounds. 'Grandad's going to be a bit slower,' my seven-year-old granddaughter was warned. 'You might notice him walking more slowly and shaking a little.' The explanation was listened with admirable attentiveness, before the wide-eyed question: 'Can you catch it?'

Presenter Dave Clark's appearances on Sky Sports were the unexpected catalyst for my sharing my news more widely in January 2018. Diagnosed with Parkinson's in 2011, he was warned that his career in front of the TV cameras would expire in just two or three years. He continued for almost ten. I knew Dave from the Capital Gold sports team, and it was inspiring to see him cope on screen, hand in pocket, but speaking normally and ploughing on with his career. I concluded that I too should speak openly, and demonstrate similarly that it is possible to continue with one's life. I need not become solely a flag-waving 'Mr Parkinson's', but the way I conducted myself could bring hope to someone else and pay back some of the debt from all that life has given me. The illness does not have to define you.

Like Dave, I try to keep my hands in my pockets; or joke about the trembling. Nevertheless, I feel tense and self-conscious when I address people in public, fearing all eyes are on me as I walk in a room. Friends usefully reassure me that my Parkinson's is not obvious; and if people do notice, it matters little. On sensible days, I concede the conceit of thinking that people are always looking at me.

'It's a real bastard,' said Chris Tarrant in his typical way. He was amongst the first to get in touch, with a hugely welcome and typically generous call. Our relationship has always been good and, knowing how well he keeps his counsel in an industry famed for its gossips, I have always been able to be honest with him. He assured me that he would help in any way he could, and troubled to follow the call with a touching handwritten note in which he pledged again to offer support. I shall never forget his kindness.

You fear too that your working life will grind to a halt, so I was delighted to hear promptly from Terry Underhill, who ran a group of commercial radio stations. I was hosting *Kid Jensen's Flashback 40* for his company, which I always found fun to do. 'I want you to know you'll always have a place here as long as I am in a position to help. I'm on your side. Don't worry about the contract.' Never before have I valued the vibe of a radio station quite so much; and I treasured the distraction of being briefly back amongst the banter as I recorded the shows in Stoke-on-Trent. In times of challenge, there is no substitute for waking up knowing you have something to look forward to.

Later, Jools Holland called to say he had just heard the news. He too promised to help in any way he could, pledging to call again in a couple of months 'to see how you're getting on'. It was touching too to receive a call from Noel Edmonds, and Steve Wright was hugely encouraging when I was interviewed on his gigantic Radio 2 programme. That appearance is still mentioned to me by listeners to this day. Love the show, Steve.

Not only is it the calls from familiar figures from radio and music that get you through, it is the lovely thoughts from people you have never met before. In the days following my announcement, over fifty thousand messages of support fell into my inbox from listeners, Crystal Palace fans and people who had just been touched by my story in some way.

I valued too the support from the research and support charity, Parkinson's UK, of which I am now an ambassador. I am also a supporter of the Cure Parkinson's Trust, which is working to fund research to slow, stop and reverse Parkinson's. There is a sense of comfort in helping others. I hoped that I could make constructive use of my public profile, just as Dave did, to heighten understanding of the condition. Its assault on the brain is not confined to older people, and that person you think is drunk as they stagger down the road at ten in the morning may not be. Billy Connolly has done much good work too, leaning on the gift he has: 'I've got Parkinson's disease... and I wish to f*** he had kept it to himself.'

Irish radio and TV presenter Gareth O'Callaghan later told me that he was on-air when he came across the *Daily Mail* article about my circumstances. He had been noticing identical symptoms and suspected something was awry, but also kept putting off any medical investigation. A doctor's appointment was made that night, and Multiple System Atrophy was diagnosed the following day. It was, of course, not news he wanted to hear but, like me, at least he could start to benefit from the necessary care and support.

My illness was part of every thought in the first days following the diagnosis, a dark shadow greeting me seconds after waking each morning. Now it occurs to me much less, although my demanding exercise regime has become a necessary part of my daily timetable, with over two hours a day of Tai chi, press ups, jogging and walking.

The medication continues alongside in earnest. Fingers are wagged, and I am warned my tablets must be taken exactly as prescribed if I am to fend off this monster as long as possible. 'Twelve o'clock means twelve o'clock – not ten-past,' insists the consultant. Accustomed to being punctual for news bulletins on-air, I rather hoped I might manage that feat.

The hallucinations continue too as the medication is faded up or down, balancing the effect of the Parkinson's and the side-effects of the pills, trying to ensure the best mix. Going to the loo at night, I meet my weird friends on the stairs, the faces unfamiliar but never scary. They seem happy to see me – and utterly real, until I reach out and put my hands through their bodies. Despite the fact I've lived through the heady days of the late '60s and '70s, and mixed in exactly the right colourful circles, I've never been much of a drug-taker, but have now discovered a little of what it might have been like.

I have not cried. Sad movies make me cry, or when my friend Ian Wright was brought off the bench at Wembley to score against Man U and put us in the lead.

Blood dripped from the gash in my forehead as I climbed into the taxi after leaving Sky TV at Isleworth. In poor light, I had fallen on climbing up the staircase from the studios after an interview. The driver kindly dispensed some tissues from his glove compartment to help mop things up, and I apologised, of course, in the most British of ways. The warnings came back to me of the most likely aggression Parkinson's might threaten. I cannot regain my balance from the sort of minor stumbles we all have from time to time.

Guðrún has been taking care of me, and little I can ever say can pay the debt I owe her for her love and care. I can think of no-one else who could have helped me as much as she has. She gets anxious about me – and annoyed when I do not do as I am told.

I do not have a bucket list. Death does not bother me, but I fear pain. Pain for me, and for my family. I do not want people to be sad. I have been upset that I may not see my seven grandchildren grow up.

I've reflected on my privileged professional life, achieving everything I dreamed of and more. I have broadcast to the whole of Europe on the mighty Radio Luxembourg, and on the national BBC Radio 1 at its zenith. I have played football with the Rolling Stones, been hugged by Elton, sat next to Princess Diana, and enjoyed the friendship of John Peel. I have watched Queen play in their earliest days and been backstage at Live Aid. I have enjoyed pop star status – just for playing the music I love.

Who could wish for more?

2.

BEGINNINGS

The basement to our white stuccoed bungalow in Vancouver was my dad's retreat. Down the stairs he strode, to retire to play his beloved jazz music, which echoed around the house. That was the music I grew up to, whether I liked it or not, played from behind a curtain in the corner of the underground room packed with treasured items from his rich life in music and radio. The walls stacked high with priceless albums and precious books; a shrine of oft-played LPs from Miles Davis and Charlie Parker, and books autographed with seemingly genuine affection from the top names. Messages with a kiss on the bottom from Billie Holiday.

In 1969, a year after I left home, my mother climbed down those stairs to his den. In an act which was totally out of character, she seized these trophies of his life and deposited them on the refuse dump in Vancouver. This was the way she chose to deal with a painful divorce from a philandering husband.

Our early home in British Columbia was typical of the era on this Pacific island. Rows of neat 1950s buildings, geometrically organised and filled with families from all around the world. Our own family included two grandmas hailing from Glasgow, and grandfathers from Denmark and Lincolnshire. Copies of the mumsy *People's Friend* magazine were delivered as a reminder of my grandparents' home and roots. I had a younger sister and a brother eight years younger than me, and we all felt closest to my mum, a registered nurse at the local hospital.

My dad broadcast on CKLG (Canada Kelowna Longshore). By day, the radio station played the music typical of the age, from Rosemary Clooney to Bert Kaempfert. By night, his more maverick two-hour programme took to the air, which was altogether more specialist. His reputation was akin to a John Peel figure on this popular station in this golden era for jazz, and musical luminaries would travel eagerly from the US to appear on the show.

For a childhood birthday, he bought me a copy of 'The Siamese Cat Song' from *Lady and the Tramp*. Whilst that novelty release became the first record I owned, rock'n'roll soon crashed into my life, heralded by the excitement of Elvis Presley rolling into town. The King rarely made appearances outside the US, and yet he was to be live in our hometown, given we had moved by this time to Vancouver. His 1957 show at the Empire Stadium was to be one of the most legendary concerts of his career, and his last-ever performance away from his home country.

CKWX was the local rock'n'roll radio station, with energetic presenters beaming out the latest hits from pioneers such as the Everly Brothers and Eddie Cochran. It was to be expected that it would adopt the Elvis concert that August night. Outside the stadium, an outside-broadcast – or remote, as we called them in Canada – was staged to mark the occasion. The streets were packed, with over 25,000 hyped-up young Canadians charging down the field from their stand to get close to the goal line where Elvis gyrated on stage.

My bedroom at home was a typical teenage den. Glued to the walls were pictures of my ice hockey heroes from the Toronto Maple Leafs, the closest team I could identify with. A tartan blanket given to me by one of my aunts from Scotland lay across the bed. But my radio was my most precious possession – a pocket-sized black and silver set with a thumbnail dial which served as my window on the world. After school, I hurried home and forsook my homework in favour of enjoying the magic of the medium as it delivered the vibrant hits of the moment.

Another rite of passage was buying my first disc from the local record store with my own pocket money. Kelowna, where we spent many holidays, boasted but a single outlet, stretching out just to the size of an average corner shop, but it dripped with vinyl and sheet music. The store was run by a young woman from England whose husband, Mark Ackerman, worked at the radio station as a commercial copywriter. At weekends as I grew older, Mark sometimes offered to drive me to Winfield, twenty minutes up the coast. En route he introduced me to music I had never heard before, and I drank in the immaculate voices of Otis Redding and Aretha Franklin, and the whole Motown sound.

Sunday night TV in North America brought the *Ed Sullivan Show*, and it was this huge variety performance which first brought the sounds of the now familiar British hitmakers to our shores, including the Beatles. Their popularity quickly grew, to the extent that boys wore Beatles wigs to school and weekend radio programmes featured excited DJs trumpeting 'Battle of the Bands: Beatles vs the Beach Boys, who is the most popular band in Vancouver right now? Call in and vote – we'll tell you who's won at six o'clock tonight.' I can recite the exact phrase even now, and little these days on radio seems, to me, to rival the magic of that sort of true radio event in the '60s.

In stark contrast to the fresh-faced all-American Beach Boys, there was something about the anarchy of the Kinks which attracted me. The stories of the brothers' battles, and the infamous onstage fight in Cardiff in 1965, when drummer Mick Avory knocked out Dave Davies with a drum pedal before fleeing the venue, fearing he had killed him. All was later smoothed over, even though Dave's wound merited sixteen stitches at the local infirmary. Not only did I like the music, I wanted to be part of the band. I did not dare to dream that, one sunny day, Ray Davies would run up behind me in Regent's Park, grab me by the waist, lift me off the ground and shout: 'You'll always be a kid to me!', before continuing his jog through the greenery. He will never quite know just how much that larking around meant to me.

Adolescents are hard-wired to strike out to define their own distinctive personality, so when bands became too popular and mainstream we had to identify edgy new idols and promptly shift allegiance. I stood up for the rootsy sound of Bob Dylan, listening incessantly to his album *Another Side of Bob Dylan*, not least the track 'Motorpsycho Nightmare', based in part on Alfred Hitchcock's movie *Psycho*. Given its nature and length, I knew few others in my peer group would trouble to listen to it. I doubt I would even have indulged in playing it in later life on my most eclectic album shows.

My taste in music was probably not the cause for me to be bullied at school. Who knows the reason? Bullies will always find one. I was shy. I was pale. 'Pinky' was my hated nickname, earned by my turning from very white in the winter to pink in the summer when my mother drowned me in calamine lotion to save my painfully pale skin from the unforgiving Canadian sun. Even now, that antiseptic smell evokes memories of those uncomfortable days.

My high school boasted its own internal closed-circuit 'radio station', which I was anxious to join. Summoning up the necessary courage one day, I knocked on the door to ask whether I might play a part. Inside it looked a little like a pirate station, with some basic facilities installed in the far corner of the room and two pupils hunched over a desk working on some project. As I joined them, a few painful seconds elapsed before one looked up and grunted: 'There is one too many of us in here.' The impact of such slights is clear when one still remembers them so vividly as an adult, yet I was not defeated – simply more determined.

One particularly annoying fellow pupil took issue with anything and everything I did. Although a friend counselled that my response should simply be to 'whack' him, violence was not in my nature. My strength was running, however, with track-and-field always my Sports Day destiny, delivering impressive times for the 220-yard race. In one memorable 440-yard run, I was way ahead of my adversary – and blessed with time to plan tactics. Typically, he used to tie his towel in a knot and lash me on the legs as I ran, but on this occasion, before he had time to strike, I nudged him and belted him with the towel myself. Taken by surprise, he stumbled and fell. It felt good. Such conduct does not sit easily with my nature, but I was never troubled again. Maybe I could have better heeded the lesson later in life with some members of radio management.

Taking advantage of my dad's radio connections when he moved across to some small city stations in the Okanagan valley in British Columbia, I managed to secure an early opportunity in the industry which was to become my life. At one local station I was taken on as a helper, with my voice first heard on-air delivering a commercial for a car company. Aged 14, I was then invited to host the teen show, stopping by on my return from school to perform enthusiastically on-air. The station boasted a large roadshow vehicle with a drop-down booth where smiley girls gave away freebies of Rothman's cigarettes – a questionable sponsorship arrangement for a teenage broadcast. With my programme sandwiched between a country music show and all manner of other random offerings catering for distinct audiences, this was genuinely traditional 'full-service' radio. Maybe jealousy of my genuine radio gig had been at the heart of the bullying.

At Capital Radio, in later life, I was invited to a glittery function at Handel & Hendrix, a curious museum in London dedicated to the lives of baroque composer George Frideric Handel and the singer-guitarist Jimi Hendrix, who had lived in adjacent Mayfair properties, separated by a wall and two hundred years. Over wine and nibbles, a woman recognised my voice from across the room and sidled over. Shaking my hand, she introduced herself as Kathy Etchingham, Jimi's girlfriend, and told me how they used to return home after clubbing and drinking, flop on the bed, and switch on my programme. Picturing that bedroom scene, with my idol clinging on to my words and the music I played, remains one of my biggest-ever career highs, although it would have been thoroughly intimidating had I been aware of the VIP listener whilst on-air. As Kathy related her tale, it passed through my mind how wonderful it would have been to call up the gang who had given me such a hard time at school to tell them that Jimi Hendrix was a fan of mine.

'Could do better' was the comment most teachers scrawled on my end of term reports. The conclusion was accurate. I was not hugely impressive on any academic front, never quite mastering the art of learning how to learn, but faring better in subjects which relied on memory.

Music study was a favourite subject, and I was tested for pitch, memory and rhythm before the violin, trumpet or saxophone were recommended as options for an instrument best-suited to my talents for the school band. The trumpet was chosen, principally on budgetary grounds as our family could not stretch to buying a saxophone. Now, I proudly possess one of these beautiful instruments. With its huge versatility, whether played softly or more energetically in a honking style, it is the ultimate instrument for jazz, a genre for which I have developed genuine affection.

○

You always remember your first serious love. Aged seventeen, I was crazy about a girl called Christine, the sort of sunny, healthy-looking brunette you might see in orange juice ads. With her lovely smile and charm, I felt the luckiest guy in the world, although the relationship was interrupted reasonably swiftly with the acute pain which first liaisons typically bring.

One afternoon, whilst thoroughly preoccupied with this latest 'bust-up', I shuffled reluctantly to class. Maths was not a subject I enjoyed, generally owing to an acute dislike of the teacher – a pipe-smoker in a baggy grey suit who left a smell of burning leaves wherever he walked. He never understood me, and seemed to have little tolerance generally of the less-gifted pupils. Halfway through this particular lesson I snapped, standing up and announcing I was leaving the classroom. He barked back that I would never be allowed back. 'Thank God,' I snarked, and departed.

There ended my schooldays, much to the concern of my mother. Only later, as a parent myself, did I really understood how the uncertainty of her son's future must have felt for her, but these were different times when schools and parents appeared to communicate rarely, and parents and children seemed to have a less equivalent relationship.

My schooldays were not traumatic; they were simply largely irrelevant. Whilst I half-heartedly mulled over fall-back careers as a marine biologist or oceanographer, indulging my love of the sea, my early experience on-air confirmed that radio would be my destiny. I felt an utter and inexplicable conviction that my mind could dream myself into that world, and I had the determination to ensure it would.

3

RADIO DREAMS

'Kelowna' is the word for a grizzly bear in the old Salish language. In Canada, the city which bore its name was the apple capital, boasting beautiful beaches on the eastern shore of Okanagan Lake, and surrounded by parks, pine forests, vineyards, orchards and mountains, and seeing less rain than Florida. Going for a long drive was a treat, speeding through the greenery by the lakes and snow resorts.

Each summer, my family used to congregate there for a couple of months to enjoy the swimming, water skiing and speed boat rides. Their beach cottage there had wisely been bought in the 1940s, at a time when they were less scarce and less expensive. In later years, Paul Rodgers of the band Free was no doubt less fortunate when he purchased a lovely property there for his family. Growing up, I relished the moments after dark when I headed down to the beach on my own, clutching my treasured transistor radio, to enjoy the sound of US and Canadian stations with their transmitters powering their signals up and down the thirty mile stretch of the Okanagan Lake.

In later years, I gravitated again to Kelowna, finding an opportunity at CKOV (Canada Kelowna Okanagan Valley). The station's sound fitted the mood of the area perfectly, with the on-air flavour of an idyllic summer holiday. Indeed, its descendant now appropriately calls itself Beach Radio 103.1.

Based off Main Street, the CKOV premises were the sort you might see in a movie set in a radio station. Like many stations in my country, its roots stretched back decades, having been established by the Kelowna Amateur Radio Club in 1928 as an amateur radio station, with the call letters 10AY.

Once through the door, we climbed the stairs to the reception area across the polished green and red patterned floor, turning left for the business end of the operation and right for the studios. Like many radio mixing desks of that vintage, the slider faders we see today were absent, and we used instead rotary knobs or 'pots' (potentiometers) to fade up the sounds from the turntables, tapes and microphones. One odd memory I have of the studio facilities is that we never wore headphones, as presenters did on every other radio station, yet the speakers puzzlingly did not 'feed-back'.

Announcers, as we called them, worked hard, and in addition their on-air duties they were required to dash out on sales appointments to bring in advertising and sponsorship deals in return for commission which formed an appreciable proportion of their remuneration. Some were salespeople first and presenters second.

At the outset, I served as a general helper, scribbling commercial scripts and generally lending an eager hand with the classical music station under the same ownership, CJOV FM. I volunteered to operate the mixing panel in the studio, before graduating to host a baroque and chamber music programme on Saturday nights called *Music for Dining*, thanks in part to some knowledge of the genre, but mostly to my ability to read record sleeve notes out loud with a deceptive degree of authority.

Accordingly, a passage from Holst's *Planets* suite came to be the first track I ever played on radio. Hearing it now reminds me of my days hosting that serious show, aged sixteen, sponsored by 'Day's Funeral Services of Kelowna'. In those times, we read our own commercials and enthused about the clients, but it would have been wholly inappropriate to repeat our office joke that the programme was more about music for dying than dining.

A tragic example of how radio touches people's lives came at CKOV. A serious car accident occurred in the city, in which two girls lost their lives instantly. One of my fellow presenters rushed into the studio to tell me about this major incident whilst I was on-air. He had driven past the awful scene en-route, and witnessed the wreckage strewn across the road and the emergency services, with lights flashing, cordoning off the area. He observed too that he could hear my voice loudly on the radio, rising from the smoking metal. Knowing that your voice was the last the victims heard is an odd feeling. You affect listeners in ways you can never imagine, and never forget an incident such as that or the families involved.

The station enjoyed an impressive standing in its community, with its announcers regarded as true local ambassadors. Not only did they visit clients, they cultivated station partnerships, participated in key events and became part of the fabric of the area. CKOV attached significant value to the equity of its on-air talent, although that did not appear to stretch to remuneration for the extra-curricular work.

Like many aspiring presenters, my voice on-air sounded high and pale, as can be witnessed by cringeworthy early recordings. Most announcers were much older than me and blessed with what was then seen as a 'DJ voice' in an era when presenters routinely lowered their voices on-air and projected in a way that is less common now.

By 1968, my role also extended to a cameo appearance on the national radio service CBC. Each week, the channel invited a local broadcaster from somewhere along the Trans-Canada highway to serve as the regional representative for the territory on its Saturday night music round-up. The programme was hosted in Toronto, and I was questioned remotely, as a contributor, about the latest local music trends and interests. Sly and the Family

Stone's *Dance to the Music* was my first Record of the Week. Like the BBC, the CBC at the time was regarded as a somewhat traditional broadcaster, but it nevertheless was a station of huge scale and I calmed myself before my coast-to-coast appearances by simply having fun and imagining a single listener, who was just like me.

In the Canadian radio market in that era, on-air talent on the many local stations were not seen as 'radio stars'. The role was regarded as just another job, or, as we said back home, we were 'a dime a dozen'. Word reached me, however, that elsewhere across the world being on radio was something more special.

By chance, I got to know a scoutmaster who had worked in radio elsewhere in the country, and was an excellent presenter. Highly-familiar with the international radio scene, he was a fund of sound advice and good ideas. Former UK pirate radio broadcaster Steve Young had also arrived at my station in 1967, and regaled me with tales of his days at Radio Caroline North, on board its rusty ship in the Irish sea in the Sixties, when he had been heard across the Midlands and north of England and much of Wales, Scotland and Ireland. Known on-air in those fun times as 'the curly-headed kid in the third row', he hosted the overnight show in a truly remarkable phase in UK radio history. Before the belated arrival of commercial radio and any BBC pop services, the pirate stations were the only place in the UK to hear the hits, and they attracted huge audiences. My energy was further fuelled by seeing an episode of the TV thriller *Danger Man* called 'Not So Jolly Roger' in 1966, filmed at Radio 390, a genuine pirate station based on the Red Sands fort in the North Sea. One of the characters in the drama pointed out, 'We don't have a licence to broadcast, a situation which worries no-one, apart from the Government.'

I pestered Steve to show me his pile of fantastic scrapbooks of the UK radio scene, overflowing with photographs and cuttings of what appeared an enviably colourful life in Sixties Britain: pictures of good-looking girls, great clothes, and radio DJs rubbing shoulders with famous faces. The country was clearly setting the trends around the world, with the energy and vibrancy of its music, fashion – and radio.

I was playing my own humble part in the music scene in Canada. Now, living away from home for the first time in an untidy house across Highway 97 in Winfield, a neighbourhood just to the north of Kelowna, with a few members of a band called Strange Movies, I acted as their manager. Whilst we still had to eke out a living pumping gas, picking cherries and delivering newspapers, there was one proud booking – a gig supporting Van Morrison's band Them at the local ice rink.

There was little by way of familial encouragement, with my dad cautioning against the risks of a career in radio: 'What makes you think you are so special?' Whilst the question might sound unkind, and our relationship was never close, he worried that a true radio gift was a prerequisite for such a competitive industry, and he could not yet see that in his son. The doubt stemmed from his own painful journey into the industry, having started out as a cab driver and sales representative with General Electric before eventually inching his way into a niche in his very specialist radio field.

In that era, securing a job in radio demanded you showcase your abilities by the submission of a reel-to-reel audition tape to the stations at which you aspired to work. I was told that they should last no longer than ten minutes, and mine lasted nine. A copy is still in my cupboard to this day, painstakingly assembled with clips illustrating my style and my voice, albeit I was trying to sound twenty years older than I was. Lovingly packaged, the reel was despatched with enthusiastic covering letters, and I waited as the parcel made its journey across the seas to prospective employers in far-off lands.

Radio Veronica was an early target for my aspirations, a hugely-popular pirate station, then based onboard the *Norderney* anchored off the Dutch coastline. The organisation had been founded in 1960 by radio dealers who believed that the existence of a pop station would boost set sales.

At Steve's recommendation, my efforts were then focussed on what was then a fledgling BBC Radio 1. That UK station had recently launched on the AM band as a spin-off from what had been the BBC Light Programme, to capture the audiences who had been sorely disappointed by the abrupt Government-imposed closure of the British offshore pirate radio stations. Although it might seem ambitious for such a callow presenter to aspire to graduate straight to a national station, there was little alternative, given the new BBC local stations were few and speech-heavy, and UK commercial music radio had yet to begin. Whilst opportunities were accordingly very few, it was that very scarcity of stations that guaranteed a major national profile for any lucky recruits.

My letter was addressed to Mark White, an imposing white-haired man with a handlebar moustache and a military bearing who was charged with helping to programme BBC Radio 1 to its huge audiences. As the grandly-titled Assistant Head of the Gramophone Records Department, he had been the conscientious producer who troubled to rewind the audition tape sent in from Ireland by a careless 28-year-old Terry Wogan, who had sent it laced backwards. Without Mark's diligence, radio history would have been notably different.

My tape was wound properly, with the correctly-coloured leader tape spliced carefully at each end, but it did not receive the same ready welcome as Terry's efforts had from the Irish broadcaster RTÉ. The typed response thanked me politely for my application, and promised to keep it on file. In the puzzling way of the BBC, Mark did suggest that they were offering programmes of fifteen minutes' duration to try-out new talent, which seemed an odd strategy to someone like me, reared on shows of three hours' duration.

My second audition tape was posted to Radio Luxembourg, the licensed European station whose English service was beamed across much of the Continent by huge transmitters on short wave and on the famous 208 wavelength on medium wave. Again, with so little music radio on offer it attracted huge UK audiences for its evening pop service programming, despite painful reception quality on transistor radios, where it faded in and out with a peculiar and very distinctive phasing sound. Indeed, the effect – caused when one AM radio signal bouncing across the ionosphere was influenced by another strong transmitter – became officially dubbed the Luxembourg Effect. The whining was tolerated willingly by listeners, and nowadays that endurance is spoken of with misty-eyed fondness.

Steve Young's dog-eared cuttings suggested to me that Radio Luxembourg presenters were stars, and I wanted to be part of that glittering scene. For me, the power of radio was clear. Listening had been a massive escape vehicle, whisking me away from the agonies of youth to a more carefree world. At night-time, the signals bounced in across the Rocky Mountains from the United States, and the intimate style of the words and music in the dark hours created a real emotional connection.

International communication in that era was a penfriend affair, so response to my application was predictably slow. Airmails were commonly used for urgent communication, with crucial messages scribbled on light blue tissue paper and flown across the world. It was a few weeks before one popped through my letterbox. Its message was stark, dictated by Radio Luxembourg's programme director, Tony McArthur.

Tony told me a job at 'Luxy' was mine – but only if I could get to Europe in ninety-six hours. My determination had paid off.

If only this penniless Canadian youth could get written parental permission… and fly across the world immediately.

4.

SWINGING BRITAIN

My large dark blue Canadian passport grandly declared 'radio announcer' as my occupation. That description was arguably not yet wholly true, but I hoped that, when I touched down at Heathrow, it would soon be.

Everything of value I had owned in Canada had been sold to fund the trip. My trumpet had gone, and my treasured blue Yahama 125 motorbike was in new hands. Like many others before and after, I arrived in this great city to build a life and reputation. My Whittington escapade to the land of cobbled streets and warm beer had to work out.

London in 1968 bubbled with energy, colour and hope. The clothes and hairstyles you see now in aged photographs were witnessed for real on the streets. Places like Carnaby Street were peppered with polka dot miniskirts, frayed bell-bottomed jeans, tall boots and long hair as the post-war generation marked out its territory with pride. In time, I was to look to Jimi Hendrix's colourful shirts for inspiration, and favoured the range by Malcolm Hall whose styles were to bless ABBA, Bill Wyman and Paul McCartney. Men's shirts boasted huge collars, almost to the extent that if the wind caught you from the front you expected to be whisked off your feet like Mary Poppins.

This characterful city was the focus of popular culture, and I penned gushing notes to friends back home in British Columbia. Just being in London was a symbol of success. They were unlikely to make the journey across, but were smitten by all they had heard about life here, just as I had been.

Aside from the forward fashion, the music scene was alive. Over the years I relished the experience of seeing the Who's first performance of *Quadrophenia*, and gigs from Eric Clapton and Cream. Clubs staged live music and the many venues thrived, from the atmospheric Whisky-A-Go-Go on Wardour Street to the Bag of Nails, Revolution and the Pheasantry, which sticks in my mind due to the occasion I bumped into Rolling Stones founder Brian Jones sitting at an adjacent table there. The profound effect of my new station on that band was made clear in Keith Richards's autobiography, *Life*, when he wrote of the records that influenced him: 'The one that really turned me on, like an explosion one night, listening to Radio Luxembourg on my little radio when I was supposed to be in bed and asleep, was 'Heartbreak Hotel'. That was the stunner. I'd never heard it before, or anything like it.'

Radio Luxembourg was part of the fluorescence of the day, a shining light in a grey post-war era. Its boss, programme director Tony McArthur, greeted me in London. Australian-born, he had been on-air himself in Luxembourg, Sydney and on-board the slickest of the pirate stations, Radio London. A lively, colourful character full of energy, ideas and enthusiasm, he was to become known for managing Shirley Bassey, Charles Aznavour and Rick Wakeman. Tony worshipped the sound of American radio, which was some way ahead of UK music radio at that time, motoring along at a whole different pace, and my North American voice seemed close enough to the sound he sought.

The innocent eyes of this eighteen-year-old Canadian boy were soon opened as I was shown around London – the city where I would really start to grow up. First stop: Soho, led by Radio Luxembourg presenter Tony Windsor. Although he never behaved inappropriately, I got the feeling that he was rather taken by me. I guess my long blond hair back then did have its appeal.

Tony Windsor – 'TW' – had also grown up in Australia, where

he had enjoyed much success before making his name in the UK onboard the pirate Radio London, not least thanks to his trademark 'He-llo' salutation, delivered in the way only he could with his booming voice. Armed with many of the tapes and contacts he had amassed whilst programming Radio London, his job at Luxembourg was to identify the sort of new talent who thrived on live broadcasting and could help the station carve out a fresh reputation, which was sufficiently 'hip' to pick up more of the pirate radio legacy audience. Alan Keen, who took up the General Manager role from Geoffrey Everitt a few months after my arrival, tells of the day he began work in his new senior management role at the station and picked up a copy of *Melody Maker* which listed what it judged to be in or out of fashion. Radio Luxembourg lay in the damning 'out' column.

TW treated me to the sort of lavish lunch I had never experienced before. From barely being able to afford meals back home, I was whisked out to the Connaught in swanky Mayfair. Waiters fussed around as this gawky teenager tried to work out in which order he should use the cutlery. Foodie Paul Gambaccini took me there again recently, and we still drew breath and remarked about the level of savings you'd need to cash in if you sought to treat someone to the full three courses and a decent bottle of wine.

As TW and I chatted, he paused and stared at my face, drawing attention to my acne, and duly dispensed some make-up cream to disguise the spots. He was an ardent fan of Cilla Black, referring to her as 'Cill', and tried to persuade me to watch her shows. I was not convinced our tastes in TV – or in many things – were likely to be compatible.

So high were my hopes for London from all I had heard and seen, I was surprised that the entire capital was not as glitzy and showbiz as I had hoped. Outside its heart, it appeared even provincial. I noticed too from the dirt under my fingernails that the air was noticeably of poor quality compared with back home.

Although significant sooty strides had been made since Victorian times, it was still much worse than today's levels, given these were the days when mountains of coal were being burned to serve heavy industry.

Radio Luxembourg's London base lay just down the road from the Connaught, at a stone-faced 38 Hertford Street. The four-storey building, now marked fittingly by a commemorative blue plaque, appeared more like a Secret Service headquarters rather than a pop station. Once through the door, visitors were greeted by a team of friendly administrative staff, and Vera Lynn's daughter Virginia, who supported the organisation in both its commercial efforts and programme production. The building also housed other business units, including the record labels they owned, becoming a beacon for the music industry with a steady flow of artists, managers and engineers coming through its doors. In my time, a young Billy Ocean was housed in the basement in his early career, writing songs for other artists before going on to enjoy six of his own UK Top Ten hits.

The walls of the Hertford Street premises were imbued with the echoes of radio and music history. Top artists such as Cliff Richard and Petula Clark had recorded their regular fifteen-minute shows for the station here in the Fifties and Sixties, as had the presenters of the time such as Pete Murray, Barry Alldis and, briefly, Kenny Everett.

Live broadcasts from Hertford Street were not permitted, for the only licensed UK broadcaster at the time was the BBC. Not only could Radio Luxembourg not transmit from Britain, it was not even allowed by the Post Office to commission landlines to convey programmes from London to the transmitters in Luxembourg. Over the years, therefore, the strategy had been to record shows in London and courier the many tapes by plane to Luxembourg for transmission. Originally recorded at a speed of thirty inches per second, as opposed to the usual high professional standard of fifteen, it was a wonder the aircraft ever took off with their heavy cargo.

The London offices boasted two studios and control rooms, well-equipped by the standards of the day with hefty EMI BTR2 tape machines, as used for recording the Beatles at Abbey Road. There were also some Philips tape recorders, coupled with two chunky Garrard 301 turntables which are now collectors' items. Another turntable was equipped to play some of the discs still coming from America using the early vertical cut method of audio recording, otherwise known as 'hill and dale', where discs were played from the inside outwards rather than resting the pick-up arm first on the outer rim, in the way which became the standard.

Whilst Studio B was restricted to 'gram programmes', where records were played, the larger Studio A allowed also for the recording of live performance. In my time with the station the likes of the Stones and Bowie used the facilities, and they were used for several legendary Monty Python albums, with gifted Radio Luxembourg producer Al Bailey on-hand. The studio benefited from large hinged pinewood blocks, which could be left in place when a 'bright' sound was desired or folded back to reveal the cushioned absorbent tiles underneath for a softer acoustic sound. In earlier days, a small ceramic tiled 'toilet', minus the lavatory facilities, had served as a convenient echo chamber.

Formula One racing driver Stirling Moss happened to live in the mews which backed onto Studio A. When a raucous act was being recorded in a late-night session, he was known to bang on the back door demanding the volume be turned down. On other occasions, if the act was to his taste he took full advantage of his proximity and popped in.

The large record library was located on the second floor, with a collection of 45s, LPs and the heavy old 78s, although the latter were quickly being discarded.

At this stage in its colourful history, Radio Luxembourg's audiences risked falling victim to the nascent BBC Radio 1, with 208 being seen less as the spiritual home for a young Brit. The programming strategy, therefore, was to modernise and make the station again the fashionable listen. A key part of this approach was to replace the recorded shows from London with more exciting and reactive programmes live from Luxembourg.

Having been fully briefed on the Radio Luxembourg operation, I began recording my first programme at Hertford Street – the *Decca Records Show*. This was a legacy concept for the station, which had long carried segments paid for by record companies simply trumpeting their own releases – of whatever quality – with little editorial oversight from the station. By the time I arrived, the programmes funded by record labels were declining, although Decca's survived for a while, remembered for the chimes of its famous D-E-CC-A jingle. I was instructed to play a one-minute clip of each track, to allow as many as possible to be included, before announcing their title, artist, producers and serial number, and then make abundantly clear the record was 'Now available from HMV'.

The strategy, therefore, was to sell records rather than please the audience. Music was selected not by a radio programmer, but by the record company which had turned down the Beatles. The new management view of such programming was clear to Alan Keen: 'I inherited a situation which to me was an embarrassment, and still is to a certain extent. That was that Radio Luxembourg permitted record companies to run this station, and I made it clear from the very offset that I was working towards the day when this selling of airtime to the record companies would end.'[1]

The Radio Luxembourg *Power Play*, introduced originally by Keith Fordyce in 1957, was an early sign of a fresh approach, where record companies paid for a single new quality song to be

1   *Deejay*, February 1973.

aired in full and highlighted straight after the news bulletins for a whole week, trumpeted by a fitting dramatic jingle. Radio ads for new records were also introduced, separated more clearly from programming editorial.

As the number of record label shows declined, Alan's commercial strategy in the early Seventies moved to a heavier reliance on traditional ad spots and sponsorships to reap station revenues. Just as with the pirates, this was an early taste of commercial radio for British youth, with campaigns for many familiar brands such as Levi jeans now heard, following deals with the major ad agencies. Unhindered by onerous British advertising rules, the station was also able to embrace cigarette and alcohol brands… and a generation can still sing the jingles for Marlboro and Peter Stuyvesant cigarettes.

Listeners in the Fifties and early Sixties will readily recall possibly the most famous advertiser of all, Horace Bachelor. Those baby-boomers can still recite the ads for his 'infra-draw' football pools winning system – delivered memorably by himself – and his address in K.E.Y.N.S.H.A.M.

Another revenue earner was the carrying of religious programming from the US. In 1953, Radio Luxembourg had been paid to broadcast the first editions heard in Europe of *The World Tomorrow* programme delivered by Garner Ted Armstrong, an American evangelist. His distinctive folksy sermons were later carried by pirate stations such as Radio London – much to Kenny Everett's annoyance – before they returned to Radio Luxembourg. Although not quite the tub-thumping of some radio evangelists, their content and style was so unusual to British ears that listeners still recognise Armstrong's name, and impersonate the programme's distinctive opening.

In due course, it was my job to pick up from the end of *The World Tomorrow* to start the station and begin my own shift on-air. Arriving in the studio one night and cranking up the loudspeaker volume, it was clear that something was amiss. One of the engineers had laced up the programme's large spool of tape the wrong way around, so that it was being played backwards on-air. With only an elementary grasp of the English language, their cursory monitoring of the output had failed to reveal the error.

Apprenticeship duly served, my months waiting in the wings at Radio Luxembourg's London outpost were over, and the time had come to move centre stage – broadcasting live to Europe from the Grand Duchy.

5

LUXEMBOURG BECKONS

The small Fokker planes which took me on my journey from Heathrow to Luxembourg Findel Airport were instantly recognisable, with their wings protruding from the top of the fuselage rather than from the side. Buckled up alone on that first hour-and-twenty-minute journey, I reflected on what lay ahead as I prepared to broadcast on what had claimed to be the world's greatest commercial radio station.

Luxembourg is a land-locked country bordered by Belgium, Germany and France, one of the smallest sovereign states in Europe. With its prosperity generated originally from steel manufacturing, it evolved into a centre for investment management. Its capital is the historic Luxembourg City, punctuated with beautiful green spaces and its famous sandstone catacombs winding on forever underground.

By good fortune, my day of arrival in the Grand Duchy coincided with fellow presenter Paul Burnett's birthday and a major party had been organised, thanks to the largesse of a German record company. Having checked into a hotel in the Place d'Armes, I joined my new team to celebrate just as they adjourned to a small club called the Chez Nous, typical of its time with a four-piece band and a range of European acts from singers to jugglers. Strippers appeared too, albeit their performance was an innocent affair by today's standards thanks to strategically placed tassels and feathers, and the lights dimming at the critical moments. Paul Burnett tells with relish the story of my introduction there to Continental life, remembering I showed up 'looking about twelve years old', wearing the sort of long furry coat with fringes which befitted the times – and fell asleep. Not only was it not particularly my scene, it had been a long day.

Radio Luxembourg was housed in the beautiful Villa Louvigny in the old town, nestling in a park of pine trees where a 'flasher' once greeted me as I walked across at night. Situated just minutes south of the city centre in the Ville Haute quarter, it was an imposing building with an eight-storey tower and porter's lodge, boasting some of the grandeur of a Royal Palace. Through the main entrance hall, a dual marble staircase complete with a statue of the Grand Duchess swept off to the left and right. Away from the showy entrance experience, offices and corridors were more functional, but there was evidence of Art Deco design, including an artistic map on the wall which bore circles pulsing from Luxembourg to signify the areas conquered by the operation's transmitters.

Although Radio Luxembourg was not a pirate station, having been on-air since 1924 and duly licensed, it shared something of the watery rebel theme, being surrounded by a moat – and something of the same disruptive spirit.

This palatial château, where the Eurovision Song Contest was staged twice in the Sixties, served as the headquarters for the station's parent company, Compagnie Luxembourgeoise de Radiodiffusion (CLR, later CLT), which operated services for many European countries in several languages on its various medium and short wave frequencies. Created in the 1920s by the enthusiastic Anen brothers with the aid of a single 50 watts radio transmitter in their attic, it grew to acquire a foothold in much of Europe because of Luxembourg's more permissive approach to commercial radio and TV station licensing compared with neighbouring lands. In the early Sixties, before Radio 1 and the pirates took hold, the station had claimed audiences upwards of fifty million listeners in more than ten different countries.

Mail arrived from all over the world in my time at the station, with a peculiar proportion of letters from Ireland, where the Luxembourg signal powered through and Irish listeners valued how we exposed some of the more contemporary acts from their fine country. There was touching response too from listeners in Czechoslovakia and Poland in those Cold War days. Western hits could only be enjoyed in those countries by buying singles on the black market or by listening to Radio Luxembourg, so those in the Eastern Bloc seemed to regard us as the voice of the free world. With their makeshift aerials, they truly valued our programmes, with one Polish listener remembering: 'A bridge towards the alternative youth cultures of the West. Radio Luxembourg allowed young people to dream their dreams and to indulge in visions of a colourful world, very much in contrast to Communism's grey and oppressive reality.'[2]

It crossed my mind that our notoriety might cause the 'authorities' to dispense with us all brutally but, as with Radio Free Europe and Voice of America, they appeared to confine themselves to occasional jamming of the signal, which was evident through a 'blip-blip' noise cutting into our programming, designed to annoy listeners to the point they would switch off. On a visit to Poland almost forty years later, a man recognised me from my voice alone and expressed his gratitude magnanimously: 'For us, you were the sound of freedom.'

We were heard everywhere, and the station's reputation was daunting, dating back to its pre-war days on long wave. I knew I was following in the footsteps of some of radio's top names and pioneers from previous generations, from Pete Murray to Keith Fordyce, and Barry Alldis to Christopher Stone, the man considered to be Britain's first disc jockey. Chris had defected to

2   Conrad Bruch: 'Remembering Radio Luxembourg in the People's Republic of Poland'.

the station in 1931, hotfoot from an angry BBC which vowed never to use his services again. Seven years later, it did.

On my arrival in 1968 I was propelled into the next generation of household names, replacing Roger Day who had left the station after just a brief spell to compere a Beach Boys tour. A former successful pirate radio name, Roger had missed the 'freedom' of Radio Caroline, and never felt comfortable at Radio Luxembourg, later recalling it as 'like the BBC with commercials.'[3]

A fresh-faced Noel Edmonds was part of the Radio Luxembourg team at the time, hugely creative and thoroughly focused on a future at BBC Radio 1. He kept his fan mail after reading it, rather than throw it away, and replied to as many letters as he could, almost as a politician would handle their constituents. Noel was not a DJ's DJ, in the sense that music was not his life. That is not to imply criticism; he simply had other priorities and was a little more of a loner, determined to carve out a very particular sort of career. We shared a keen interest in cars, and he once went for a spin in a kit car he had assembled, only to crash promptly into another vehicle at an intersection near the Villa. He was released unharmed after a hospital check-up.

Usually, life in the Villa was more about laughter. Many elaborate japes were planned, the inevitable result of throwing a group of often-bored young guys together in a large 'Big Brother' house far away from home. Ours was the first generation of Radio Luxembourg presenters who were required to make their lives in the country rather than record programmes remotely, and that spirit and comradeship could be heard on-air just as had been the case with the offshore pirate presenters confined to their ships. We were blood brothers – members of the biggest band in Europe.

On one occasion, when Noel was seeking revenge after a minor conflict with station manager John Barter, some fish was

3   www.davidlloydradio.com/conversations.

mischievously Sellotaped under John's desk. As the pungent smell grew intolerably, John threw open the large windows in disgust and asked whether anyone else could smell it. As part of the ruse all denied it, to the extent that the two English service administrators, Josie and Paula, had to rush off to hide their tears of laughter.

Another rigorously-planned hoax, featuring a knife and tomato ketchup, was staged to suggest that Tony Prince had killed his wife. I was flattered to be the butt of such jokes on several occasions, yet it never echoed with the bullying of my schooldays. If the guys at Radio Luxembourg troubled to play a joke on you, you were clearly part of the family.

Families have characters, and our era boasted many amongst its presentation team. 'Your Royal Ruler' Tony Prince was probably the closest thing to a popstar, having been lead singer of a Lancashire band called the Jasons in the late Fifties. As a vocalist and guitarist then club DJ, and Elvis enthusiast, Radio Caroline was his first port of call. Having left the ship as the stations were outlawed, he joined Radio Luxembourg in 1968 and served for sixteen loyal years, eventually rising to the post of programme director. Not the tallest of guys, he carried off with aplomb what looked like an overgrown Beatles haircut.

Worthing's Dave Christian, six feet tall and sporting dark long hair and sideburns, was new to radio, save for his efforts on a very low-powered fleet radio station in his Navy days. As a committed radio enthusiast, he got to know some pirate radio presenters at his discos on Worthing Pier and signed up to Radio Luxembourg, aged 19, at about the same time I did, exploring his passion for classic rock and soul music. Dave went on to commercial radio in Portsmouth and sadly died in 2010.

Mark Wesley joined us in 1971, another former pirate presenter and record plugger. A Luxembourg pin-up, he was musically gifted, which is where his heart really lay. He emerged, in time, as a successful copy writer, jingle-maker, songwriter, record producer and action thriller author.

Powerful-voiced Bob Stewart was encouraged to try radio presentation at the suggestion of ex-Beatles drummer Pete Best. Bob was known for the puzzle of his utterly convincing yet wholly invented mid-Atlantic accent, having been born and brought up in Liverpool. His sonorous voice shook your Hi-Fi speakers as he boomed out the familiar dramatic announcements when closing-down the station at night: 'The world's biggest independent commercial radio station, with an omni-directional power of one million 200,000 watts. Goodnight – and good morning – wherever you may be.'

On arrival in Luxembourg, I lodged briefly with Tony Prince and his wife Christine in their large ground floor apartment, sharing a room with Bob Stewart. We were unlikely roommates. As we settled in and unpacked before dinner, Bob set out the rules, instructing me not to touch him when he was asleep. 'If you touch me and I wake up, I start swinging.' To this day, I am unsure what he had expected of me – or what might once have happened to him. He later moved to the safety of his own accommodation with his wife and children.

Bob and I went out for drinks one night with John Lodge and Justin Hayward from the Moody Blues. As conversation turned to shared interests, it was clear that they loved cars as much as Bob did. When the topic of the Rolls Royce arose, Bob became dewy-eyed with enthusiasm, prompting the guys to suggest they could get him one. When he protested the state of his finances, they reminded him of their influence and indicated a deal could be done through their contacts. Next day, we hurried down the drive into the car park of the Villa Louvigny to see an area marked out for the grand vehicle, but nothing more. Until Bob caught sight of the small Matchbox toy car placed in the centre.

It was easy to see why Ben Sherman shirt-wearing Bob was the victim of such plots. When the 1973 Eurovision Song Contest was staged at the Grand Théâtre de Luxembourg, about three kilometres from the Villa Louvigny, Bob became curiously obsessed with rumours that terrorists would seize the opportunity to take control of Radio Luxembourg. A whip-round was rallied to purchase a thick rope, so that if we were in danger on the third floor, we could make our escape. He even thoughtfully placed climbing gloves alongside the coiled rope, ready for our descent, untroubled by the fact that most of us were wholly unfit and incapable of even scaling the window ledge. The precautions proved unnecessary, and Luxembourg carried off another victory with 'Tu Te Reconnaîtras', performed by the French singer Anne-Marie David.

On the historic night of the Moon-landing in July 1969, Bob and I did what everyone not watching the TV coverage that night did – we went out to gaze up in wonderment at the Moon, just to pause for a moment to wallow in the once-in-a-lifetime thought that there were people wandering about up there. As Neil Armstrong descended his ladder on to the lunar surface, we took the small steps up ours to the very top of the Villa Louvigny's turret just to feast the senses, away from the distractions, and feel seemingly as close as we could be to the incredible feat and bask in Mankind's pride.

Curly-haired Peter Powell was on the team, nursing an unlikely ambition – he wanted to be an agent representing celebrities. After progressing to a successful spell at Radio 1 after his five years at Luxy, he was to realise his specific dreams absolutely, becoming one of the best in his field as founder-chairman of the James Grant Media Group, representing top notch talent such as Ant and Dec, Simon Cowell and Davina McCall. People respect Peter; and he chooses now not to be nostalgic about his on-air days. I gather many have sought to tempt him to appear at retro gigs or on-air and all have been disappointed, no matter how generous the rewards proffered.

I was just eighteen and the kid of the bunch, to the extent that the wonderful Paul Burnett affectionately referred to me as 'Kid'. Given, in those days, there was concern about how listeners would distinguish between Dave Christian and me, Paul suggested that I ditch the name David and adopt 'Kid'. The moniker was to stick with me for much of my career, and by mid-1969 the official newspaper programme listings were already using it. Thankfully, we all chose to ignore Noel's further suggestion of calling me Foetus Jensen.

Paul Burnett and his wife Nicole were hugely supportive during my early days in Luxembourg, treating me as a stray they had discovered on their doorstep and taken in. For Paul, an only child, I was almost the kid brother he never had.

He had arrived at the station from pirate radio and Manx Radio in 1967. Not the tallest of guys, he welcomed the Seventies' fashion for towering platform shoes, and was disappointed when we all started wearing them too. As fashion statements for guys who were supposed to be on trend they were essential, but as we found as we waddled through the office as if on stilts, they had serious limitations as footwear.

Radio Luxembourg's English service was accessed by walking under the TV studios, down a corridor and up in a lift to the floor above the German and French services. Its studios were basic affairs, and throughout my whole spell at the station, presenters were not trusted to operate their own mixing desk and play in their own records, as was routine at many music radio stations around the world by that time. Instead, we sat alone in a booth at an odd-shaped decorous table, the surface of which was challenging to use for writing, with the Telefunken microphone dangling from the ceiling in front of us.

On one occasion, whilst I was reading the news, mischievous Paul Burnett twanged back the mic on its cabling, so it swung across the studio away from my mouth. I ran around the studio in pursuit of it whilst trying to continue delivering the bulletin. Poker-faced, Paul tried to convince our new arrival Dave Christian, watching, that this messing-around accounted for Radio Luxembourg fading in and out on listeners' transistor radios.

Through the large window behind us lay the park below. On warm days, we threw open the windows for ventilation and could sometimes hear people below shouting up, their cries thankfully never aired thanks to the quality of the directional microphone. Through the other window, in front of us, our technical operator could be seen in the relative darkness of the adjacent control room. They were charged with playing in the discs or tapes at our direction, although staff frequently did not speak English, so gesticulation was the lingua franca. To signal you wanted the microphone turned off when you had finished speaking, you drew your index finger across your throat, leaving a noticeable red line across your gullet after each show.

The control room was equipped with aged industrial-looking black equipment. The tape machines played the old reel-to-reel quarter-inch tape, laced on spools which lacked the luxury of the top plate they were to be sensibly given in later years to keep the tape safe on its hub. When editing a crucial interview, it was commonplace to return to your studio after an interruption to find that your tape, for whatever reason, had escaped from its housing and become an irretrievable tangle of spaghetti on the floor.

The English service on Radio Luxembourg was purely a nocturnal affair. Its broadcasts were confined to evenings, picking up from the Dutch service at 7.00pm and broadcasting until 3.00am, when we closed down with the haunting ballad 'Maybe the Morning' by US jazz vocalist Marion Montgomery. Whilst a part-time radio station might seem an odd concept, it was accepted in those times, not least because the only other pop outlet, BBC Radio 1, closed-down and handed over to easy-listening Radio 2 in the evenings. So at night, whether staying in and going out, Luxy was the soundtrack of choice for young Brits. When they were having fun, we were part of it.

Presenters surfaced at Villa Louvigny around 4.00pm, barging through the tall doors into the open-plan area. Here, we assembled for any necessary updates by phone from the boss Tony McArthur or his successor Ken Evans back in London, some discussion with John Barter, or caught up on any other admin before the office staff departed and the building metamorphosed from the business of the day to the fun of the night.

I first surfaced live on Radio Luxembourg in a range of general programmes, with the mid-January 1969 schedule showing me hosting 9.00-10.30pm, surrounded by Tony Prince, Alan 'Fluff' Freeman and Noel Edmonds. In the press listings and early photograph cards, I was referred to as 'Dave Jensen', although I do not recall using 'Dave' on-air. In that respect, I am like Pink Floyd guitarist David Gilmour, who pulled me aside at one gig I was compering to make sure I never repeated the error of calling him Dave, as I had in a soundcheck.

'All Along the Watchtower' by Jimi Hendrix was the first track played by this Canadian in Europe. There was no Radio Luxembourg presentation rule book, with its instinctive informality contrasting with a BBC still wrestling with the seismic changes the Sixties had thrust upon it. The mid-evening programmes featured the usual fresh hits of the day, from Scott Walker to the Casuals, and sometimes included *Bingo Scoop* where I was instructed to read out the numbers in the time-honoured fashion, heralded by a jingle made from Dave Carey's 'Bingo Bingo (I'm in Love)'. Radio Luxembourg had a long-standing reputation with such games, including the postal one, operated in conjunction with the magazine *Titbits*.

Management feedback on my on-air performance was sometimes delivered by Tony McArthur, usually measured and positive, and no presenter left a conversation with him feeling terrible – surely the mark of a good boss. Even as managers changed, they valued the talent they had inherited, and we did not feel the vulnerability UK presenters now feel on regime changes. Whilst the company was successful in generating revenues, we did not feel hostage to the next set of audience figures or over-anxious to create the next big stunt or contest. I did not feel the destructive atmosphere of criticism I was to experience on occasions in my later career. Maybe it sounds just a little 'hippie' to suggest that the Luxembourg approach of its day seemed to be less about the station always striving to be the hero, and more about just playing the songs.

In an interview with *Deejay* magazine in July 1973, I said: 'You have to project some sort of personality and ultimately the listener will regard you as being a friend – some sort of friend on the radio that they can turn to and trust that they are gonna hear good music.'

General manager, later managing director, Alan Keen also flew over from the London office to address us as a presentation team. He was highly-regarded for his energy and great sense of humour, not least when he and Paul Burnett were sparring. Seen as a maverick from his days pioneering pirate Radio London, he could change gear with ease and talk the language of business more conservatively when the need arose. On one occasion, he declared that he had been listening-in all week and had one comment: 'Some of you are talking too much; others are talking too little.' He looked and me and illustrated the point. 'Kid, if you're growing tomatoes, I want to know about it. We are interested.' The sound advice on the value of giving listeners a judicious degree of insight into your life was to be repeated later in my career. Alan was much-loved, and died in 2019, aged 91, just weeks after his wife.

The arrival of one of the large riveted dark blue cases from 'home' was warmly welcomed. Opening the regular consignments from England felt like being a kid on Christmas morning. We all looked forward to lifting the lid to reveal all manner of goodies, from a few national newspapers and the music trade press to packets of tea and sausages. Items from record companies arrived, via our London office, and I cringe when I think how much we took for granted and quickly discarded or gave away, from a Beatles ash tray to artist-branded T-shirts. An acetate of the 'Get Back'/'Don't Let Me Down' single from the Beatles' Savile Row office arrived, but I tossed it quickly aside thinking I would be sent a proper pressing soon. A flexi-disc of George Harrison hosting a Beatles Christmas special was similarly disregarded. I wince now when I think of the value collectors would attach to that ephemera.

The station boasted significant scale, with a Gallup poll suggesting it reached 3.6m UK listeners nightly in 1970, including the vast majority of sixteen to twenty-year olds. A station survey in Scandinavia suggested it reached 40% of people. Such was its stature, the biggest names in music ventured across to see us to gain exposure for their new releases, not least if they felt we might embrace their track as a personal 'hit pick'.

A host of clever acts dominated the music of the early Seventies, including the likes of Roxy Music. The whole thrilling band dropped by to promote their earliest albums, including Brian Eno, the colourful sax player Andy Mackay and, complete with eye make-up, Bryan Ferry. Although their distinctive art-rock image is particularly well-remembered, they were also notably great musicians. Midway through the interview, Ferry paused, then reached into his bag and pulled out a decent bottle of red wine and some paper cups. I looked on, puzzled, from the other side of the desk. After some degree of ceremony, he handed me one and held his own up to toast. 'Here's looking at you, Kid,' he said. 'I've always wanted to say that.' Owing to audience requests, Roxy's 1972 debut album *Roxy Music* was to spend many weeks in my *Hot Heavy 20* chart, which was published in *Sounds* magazine, and then on to critical acclaim and commercial success.

Other 'orders from the bar' during interviews included red wine for Al Stewart, and sherry for Rod Stewart when he visited during his days with the Faces, another one of the characterful bands I would love to have been part of. Slim Steve Harley from Cockney Rebel, with his ruffled blond hair, visited during 1973. A very entertaining man with a passion for music. Upon learning of my heavy cold, he decided to come up and see me – equipped with a bottle of cognac – and offered to massage my shoulders during our conversation. Even when ill, I was mindful that interviewees generally respond best when you go with the flow, so I accepted.

Maggie Bell, lead vocalist with the Scottish band Stone the Crows, suggested a meal and a wee dram before our live late-night chat on Radio Luxembourg. Whilst she was great company, I drink alcohol so rarely that it pounces on me revengefully. On-air later the tables were turned, with Maggie sitting up close and almost interviewing me, holding me tight to avoid my toppling over.

Record companies, too, were regular visitors as they plugged their product, and football matches between their representatives and a team from Radio Luxembourg became a regular event, with me playing in midfield.

The pluggers relished their trips to Luxembourg, with staff from Decca, CBS, Epic and couple of indie labels assembling in a noisy rabble at Heathrow before flying over en-masse. Once in Luxembourg, a custom at these get-togethers was the 'relay dinner', where the record companies, the Luxembourg DJs and their partners gathered at seven o'clock to begin eating and drinking. Every few hours, one DJ left the table to go to present their programme dutifully, and the previous one returned. As the whole evening's hospitality was paid for on their expenses, our noisy outings proved popular with local restaurants.

Having played Bowie's incredible 'Space Oddity' endlessly after its original release just ten days before the real-life moonwalk in 1969, it was good to meet the man who had written the eerie masterpiece aged 22. He visited to promote *The Man Who Sold the World*, the album which originally put aside one controversial cover design in favour of another, where he appeared reclining on a chaise longue in a cream and blue satin dress. On his trip to the studios he appeared funny, sardonic, very educated, never looking-down on people... just fighting the good fight from inside a box of eyeliner. Save perhaps for his later work with Tin Machine, I found all his studio work and his stagecraft of outstanding quality.

Around the time his fourth studio album *Hunky Dory* was released in 1971, Bowie made the trip to Luxembourg to promote what became his breakthrough work. Given our interview would be conducted live, late in the evening, he asked for ideas to kill a few hours before appearing, insisting that if we stayed in his hotel he might just drink a little too much to be coherent on-air later. I suggested exploring town and visiting the Blow Up Club, about ten minutes away, which had emerged as a credible local music venue.

On returning to the station for the programme, I innocently hopped in a cab with him. The door slammed and he nudged closer to me on the back seat. And then closer still. 'You do know I'm bi, don't you,' he said. 'I'm bicycle. Bi-weekly. Bi-lateral. And the list went on, making abundantly clear what was really on his mind. We quickly but amicably established I had little interest in bicycles – or indeed anything else bi.

On-air that night, as the interview concluded, he thanked me for having him on, 'and for taking me for a Blow Job.' A faux apology with a knowing grin was offered as the track played: 'I didn't think it would cause a problem.' My career flashed before my eyes, but he was right. It was never mentioned by anyone.

Fellow presenter Bob Stewart had a similar Bowie awakening. After a few drinks together as the city closed for the night, they had retired to Bob's apartment to continue the conversation. When Bowie remarked that Bob's furniture was 'sumptuous', stocky Bob in his lumberjack shirt soon realised that maybe they were not quite going to be as suited as he had hoped. I reassured Bob that Bowie was just being typically theatrical. Bob, however, was from fighting country, and remained a little more sceptical.

Our paths crossed again in 1973 at the Château d'Hérouville, the 18th century castle near Paris equipped with studios which Elton John had recommended to Bowie. The album *Pinups*, on which he put his stamp on the work of other artists such as the Who and the Yardbirds, was being recorded. Although he was dressed from the usual Bowie wardrobe, it was fascinating to witness him in a non-performance, toned-down mode, not preening himself in front of an audience, but working with colleagues who knew him well. He had always been confident of his own abilities, even in his earliest career when working alongside musicians a lot older than he then was. Watching him in the studio before the interview, the mood was quiet and professional, demonstrating the seriousness with which he and his band took their music.

The session came just a couple of weeks after his surprise announcement on-stage at the Hammersmith Odeon that it was 'the last show we'll ever do', and his management company issuing a statement confirming that he was 'leaving the concert stage forever'. When I asked about his plans, he suggested that he had not thought things through in detail, but he was planning to create space to pursue other things, potentially acting in films. He also spoke briefly about 'Space Oddity', suggesting it was a riposte to the glib way that the extraordinary space ventures were being portrayed by the media.

○

The Grand Duchy of Luxembourg, to give the country its full name, had been a founder member of the Common Market in 1957 and, by my time there, people were starting to travel around more freely. It was an affluent, expensive place to live, and it was not unusual to meet people who chose to live in a neighbouring country and cross borders to work. The city was sedate, a quietly confident place, and certainly one of fine restaurants and wines rather than junk food. At my tender age I failed to recognise the calibre of the cuisine when we dined out, distracted by the company and the experience – whilst drawing attention to ourselves by being the noisiest table.

US marines were a familiar sight, stopping over on their return from the war in Vietnam to give their minds much-needed time to adjust before venturing home to their families. As fellow English speakers we tended to mix socially, and Radio Luxembourg presenters were often invited to host Friday night gigs at their air base. Paul Burnett warned me to be cautious about the vicious alcohol shots called 'after-burn' we were invited to down. Short-haired and extremely fit, the Marines were nevertheless often vulnerable from their experiences, and were watched over by the sort of jar-headed guy you did not mess with, with muscles in places you did not think possible. On occasions, Marines called at the radio station, where we generally tried to be hospitable, even when one likeable guy sat by me in the studio as I read the news, throwing his knife at the wall, cutting deep into the acoustic panelling.

Luxembourg was a key destination for Iceland Air and Freddie Laker. Charter flights touched down, full of groups of girls on weekend holiday packages, so the city was most unlike the Orkney Islands in 1979 when I visited with producer Dave Tate for two special Radio 1 programmes marking the moment when North

Sea oil began to flow into Britain. With little female company, guys would slow dance with guys.

Like first love, your first proper radio station is always a fund of fond memories which are unlikely to be equalled. It is a privilege making radio, simply spending time with people of a similar age just having fun doing what you love.

One tragic incident sticks in my mind from my spell there. One of the 'speakers', as they called the presenters on the German service, took his life whilst I was on-air just feet away.

Such was the effectiveness of the sound insulation in my studio that the crack of the shotgun was not heard by me or by listeners. Arriving at work the next day, I found the police conducting a forensic examination of the cordoned-off hallway just adjacent to the English service, and I was questioned about what had happened. These sorts of tragic events are never forgotten, and leave so many unanswered questions.

After a spell living with Noel Edmonds and other colleagues, I settled into a modern apartment block on the Côte d'Eich in northern Luxembourg, on the way out of town, just as you slipped into third gear on the thoroughfare to Germany. Mark Wesley used to offer me a lift to and from the station as I had yet to pass my driving test, having relied on my old motorbike back home. Paul Burnett, who lived on the same road, obliged too, although such was the odd design of his Mercedes sports car I was squeezed sideways into the back.

Over the years my accommodation was shared with a variety of people with connections to the station, including Golly Gallagher, who was one of its live club DJs, and still a friend to this day. Paul Burnett helped me move in, although I claimed in *Fab 208* magazine that he promptly forgot which apartment I had adopted so that when he and his wife Nicole popped around with a surprise fondue, they bounded into the quiet French family's front room below.

Despite the scale of the station's audience, Luxy presenters were not heroes in the city of Luxembourg itself as our principal audience lay abroad, but when returning to the UK our growing profile was evident. Alongside John Peel, I was invited to host Pop Proms at the Royal Albert Hall in July 1969. The gig came just days after Pink Floyd's disruptive Final Lunacy gig, following which they were banned from ever appearing at the venue again after a night of smoke bombs, exploding cannons and a crew member in a gorilla suit. The ban was quietly forgotten just a few months later.

In career terms, that Pop Proms signalled my first proper gig, introducing the Equals, Marmalade and Amen Corner with Andy Fairweather Low. The night began in a promising fashion when the promoter, Harvey Goldsmith, suggested casually that we were to use the PA system belonging to the Rolling Stones as it was already installed for a subsequent performance. Looking around at the crowd of over five thousand concertgoers spread over six levels of seating, it was a far cry from lonely remotes in car parks back home in Kelowna.

Throughout my career, I went on to introduce hundreds of live acts. It was always a great feeling hearing the crowd's reaction as I walked on stage each time, although the approbation belonged really to the anticipation of the band to follow. One of my friends counselled 'enjoy the applause, but don't believe it.'

My on-air programmes developed their reputation. More and more artists readily appeared as late-night guests, and I got to know them better to the extent that we used to retire to my apartment after the interview to have a drink and chew the fat into the small hours. Johnny Nash popped in, as did Status Quo and Colin Blunstone from the Zombies. The list of late-night callers reads like an impressive Who's Who of music, but the visits were simply a pragmatic solution to a problem caused by a late programme finish and the lack of convenient flights out of

Luxembourg.

Singles chart-topper Suzi Quatro was then carving out a huge reputation down Devil Gate Drive as a woman in a male-dominated rock world, and attributed some of that success to us: 'With the release date looming, we had the radio on non-stop so as not to miss one single airing of 'Can the Can'. Radio Luxembourg played it first, and as we sat glued to the radio it sounded fantastic.'[4] Suzi was the first female bass player to become a major rock star, renowned for the leather gear she sported. She was another visitor to my flat, and, for reasons unknown, we posed together on the back of a Harley Davidson for a photo-opportunity.

The night Ronnie Wood from the Stones stopped by, he mentioned that Ian McLagan, or 'Ian Mac' as he called him, the keyboard player with the Faces, did a great impersonation of me. Sitting next to me, Ronnie phoned him and said: 'I've got Kid here – do your impression.' I concede his performance was annoyingly accurate.

My neighbours seemed to not bat an eyelid at these current or future icons wandering in and out late at night, and chose to ignore the noise we routinely made behind the sturdy blackout shutters, a feature of so many Luxembourg properties.

Aside from the glitterati, it was a typical bachelor flat, with flatmates coming and going, friends staying over and all the dubious dalliances and dodgy domesticity you would expect of guys let loose in early adulthood. Little wonder that Radio Luxembourg DJs found little favour as tenants with local letting agencies and landlords.

One irregular feature of that fourth-floor flat was the rusty old bedframe propped up on the front balcony. We had taken it out whilst moving furniture around but struggled to get it back in, so

4 *Unzipped: The Original Memoir* by Suzi Quatro.

it was left outside, with the mattress simply thrown on the floor inside. To this day, Paul Burnett still tells of how he used to smile at the incongruous landmark in this beautiful part of town as he drove by on his way to the radio station.

6

A DARK HISTORY

The faded graffiti on the walls of the caves beneath Radio Luxembourg's home told a sombre story far removed from its showbiz reputation. Each mark denoted the pain of a day in captivity for a prisoner. In my time, visitors were always eager to see the fascinating remnants of this era, including these former cells and escape tunnels.

The Villa Louvigny had been built in 1920 on a site of the 17th century fortress of Luxembourg. By 1932, it was being rented by Compagnie Luxembourgeoise de Radiodiffusion for its radio operations, and the company later bought the premises before extending them in the 1950s.

The atmosphere inside was austere. We entered by the side entrance, near the bridge over the moat, pushing open a door so heavy it took both hands to shift. Only the most special of visitors were deemed worthy of using the lofty front entrance headed by the RTL carved crest featuring the proud Luxembourg insignia, inscribed *Alas Leoni Dedit* – He gave wings to a lion.

As war broke out, the station stopped broadcasting at the request of the Grand Ducal government with broadcasts switched initially to continuous orchestral music interrupted by announcements. Then, the staff were made redundant and German troops seized the station, an invaluable asset for propaganda chief Joseph Goebbels as the powerful transmitters, with their 600 feet tall masts on Junglinster Plain, could be incorporated into the Reichs-Rundfunk-Gesellschaft to dispense Nazi propaganda.

Famously, this included relaying speeches from William Joyce, later hanged for treason at Wandsworth prison. He had been born in New York to an Irish father and English mother, moving later to Ireland. The epithet 'Lord Haw Haw' was given to him, and those like him, by a *Daily Express* journalist owing to the drawling nasal voice. Joyce and his wife worked briefly at the Villa itself during the heavy bombing of 1943/44.

Beamed to Britain and listened to by many, his sneering broadcasts were aimed to unsettle, although they were routinely so outrageous many listeners regarded them as comical. The BBC, on behalf of the Ministry of Information and the social research organisation Mass Observation, undertook research in 1940 which concluded that two thirds of adults in the UK tuned in regularly or occasionally – the same proportion listening regularly to the BBC News. Fifty-eight per cent of those questioned listened in 'because his version of the news is so fantastic that it is funny.'[5]

'Germany calling. Germany calling. The British Ministry of misinformation has been conducting a systematic campaign of frightening British women and girls about the danger of being injured by splinters from German bombs. The women have reacted to these suggestions in alarm by requesting their milliners to shape their spring and summer hats out of very thin tin plate which is covered with silk, velvet or other draping material.'

Broadcasting principally from Berlin via the transmitters of Reichsender Hamburg, Joyce recorded his broadcasts at various locations, and was said to have used a large Neumann microphone. Even now, that German brand is renowned for excellence around the world.

Propaganda also included the broadcasting of interviews with POWs, in which they were forced to give answers to suit the purpose of their interrogators. Some cleverly offered seemingly innocuous, yet incongruous responses, which were easily

5   'The Rise and Fall of Lord Haw Haw': Imperial War Museum.

identified by people back home as having been given under duress. In one poignant recording, we heard the voice of a pilot who had been shot down. One can only wonder what was have going through his head as he spoke into a microphone.

These broadcasts were recorded on huge transcription discs, noteworthy as the needle was placed on the inside to begin to replay the material, not the outside. Many of them still cluttered up the offices during my time, with the admin staff, Paula and Josie, weaving their way around them to get to their desks. Some presenters realised their significance and took one for safekeeping; others are now deposited in the British Library.

The liberation of Luxembourg began in September 1944, although Radio Luxembourg still lay vulnerable as the enemy had made plans to detonate explosives at the main transmitter. Thankfully, intelligence from the Resistance served to ensure those efforts were sabotaged. Although the building had been plundered, the station's collection of 'gramophone records' was retrieved early in January 1946 alongside other useful items, having been stored in about fifty large wooden crates kept safe in a depository in Luxembourg town and wisely moved around from time to time.[6]

As the building was reclaimed by US troops, it was reported by the US magazine *Life* that surrendering Wehrmacht soldiers even hoped to find a job if Radio Luxembourg returned. What was certainly true was that early Magnetophon reel-to-reel tape recorders were found which had been used for recording and playing out propaganda and other programming on relay transmitters. The Germans had made huge quiet advances in this field during the war, developing AC tape bias which improved the sound quality by reducing background hiss. Bing Crosby and Les Paul were quick to identify the potential from these new

---

6 'Stephen Williams and Radio Luxembourg'; Roger Bickerton, available at www. suttonelms.org.uk/articles69.html.

developments, and made early use of the technology for future commercial music recordings which had hitherto been made direct to disc.

It was always sobering to think of the stark contrast between the Villa's reputation as a home for European entertainment and its dark past illustrated by its legacy in the building. The old cells were being used for storage; some of the valves in the equipment still bore the Nazi insignia, and some of the AEG Telefunken equipment remained, still providing good service. Aged photographs show the guards on duty outside the locked gates in their familiar uniforms bearing the SS eagle insignia, with a swastika flying close by.

After liberation, the transmitters were repaired within four days and swiftly re-purposed. Propaganda was then transmitted in the opposite direction by the Anglo-American Psychological Warfare Division of the Supreme Headquarters Allied Expeditionary Forces to undermine German soldiers' morale.

On 12th November 1945, with the words 'Bonjour le Monde, ici Radio Luxembourg' the station was back, resuming English commercial programming on long wave the following year, with Stephen Williams rejoining the station from the BBC as Director of English programmes. He hired Geoffrey Everitt, who had served as an army officer in Luxembourg in the final few months of the War. Geoffrey succeeded Stephen as General Manager, and was still in post by the time I was appointed.

Few wavelengths of radio stations around the world are as famous as 208 metres; the three digits alone imbued with memories. 208 came into use for Radio Luxembourg in 1951, from a new transmission site at Junglinster, later boosted by facilities in Marnach in the north-east of Luxembourg.[7] As rock'n'roll was born, Radio Luxembourg was poised to own British audiences.

7 *The Voice of Europe* by Philip Champion; *The Radio Luxembourg* story by Nathan Morley.

WHISKEY IN THE JAR

The wistful first eponymous album from a new band called Thin Lizzy appealed instantly to me when it arrived on my desk at Radio Luxembourg. The impressive vinyl would lead to a family friendship, and ultimately tragedy.

This brilliant example of songwriting was delivered to me by Frank Rodgers at Decca, whose belief in the band was not echoed by the record company itself, which chose to offer scant organisational support for the release. At that stage, Thin Lizzy were more of a Celtic rock act rather than the one they eventually became, and only John Peel and I even entertained playing such material on radio. John had met them when they came over to the UK from Ireland on the boat to record the first album, but did not then choose to feature it heavily on his programme.

I championed that 1971 album, appointing it the Number One album on my *Hot Heavy 20*. That level of international exposure came as something of a surprise to the young band members as they drove around on tour in their white Transit van. Guitarist Eric Bell, one of the founder members, said: 'One night, we were in Ireland doing a few gigs, and some guy came up to us… and asked if we'd heard Kid Jensen playing our album. They said he was talking about it all the time on *Jensen's Dimensions* on Radio Luxembourg. He was raving about the album. He was about the only guy that was.'[8]

8   www.recordcollectormag.com: 'Bell Rings Out' by Rich Davenport.

Thin Lizzy had got together in late 1969, when Eric Bell moved to Dublin and met Phil Lynott and drummer Brian Downey at a local gig. They were later joined by Gary Moore, a friend of Eric's.

In the light of my enthusiasm for their eloquent work, Frank Rodgers at Decca brought their tall principal songwriter, lead vocalist and bassist Phil Lynott out to spend the weekend in Luxembourg with us. Our chemistry was instant, and after a little sight-seeing we adjourned to my flat in town at lunchtime. Drinks were requested, and I managed to track down a bottle of whisky but could not find any mixers. Phil suggested the use of milk as a substitute, which we duly added. I remember little of the remainder of that visit.

Phil eventually grabbed a cab to the airport, without troubling to check whether he had sufficient Luxembourgish francs in his wallet to pay the fare. Realising his predicament too late, the driver was asked to wait whilst he rushed into departures to pick out a likely looking young couple who might sympathise with his plight. Such was his charm, they put their hands in their pocket and gave him the cash he needed.

That weekend was forever referred to by us as 'the lost weekend in Luxembourg' with a mutual knowing smile, although the visit was the overture to a life-long relationship in which a quiet, softly-spoken musician turned into a swaggering, impressive frontman.

The Country Club in Middlesbrough was where I first witnessed Phil and the band on stage, and they impressed. After the gig, in March 1971, my then girlfriend and I, pursued by Decca's Frank Rodgers in his car, drove across to Manchester on the promise of joining in a late-night drinks session at a curious hotel run by Phil's mother, Philomena. As we drew up in what seemed like a quiet residential street, there were no obvious signs of the Clifton Grange Hotel. Knocking at the door of the address we had been given, a detached property with a large extension set back from the road with a small lawn, we were admitted on mentioning

Phil's name, but could hear no evidence of any party. Then, as an inner door was thrown open, a gush of noise and revelry greeted us, as if a scene change on a TV drama. It transpired that such celebrations were commonplace at the venue, which had been considerately and efficiently soundproofed.

The Clifton Grange Hotel, nicknamed The Biz, had become something of a local institution, frequented and loved by the showbiz circle in the north and commemorated in a dedicated track on Thin Lizzy's debut album. Whenever he was gigging anywhere near, Phil frequently returned to visit his mother's establishment, inviting all his friends to descend on the hotel for a huge party, including me. Those noisy get-togethers consolidated the bond between me and his family. I got the impression that Philomena valued the support I had given her much-loved son, who had never seen his Guayanan father. He had been born out of wedlock and, aged 18, his mother was thrown into a Birmingham home for unmarried mothers in those judgmental times, before settling in Manchester, which she grew to love.

That autumn we arranged for Thin Lizzy to perform in our favourite Luxembourg haunt, the Blow Up Club, on a bill headlined by the Faces.

The band's second album, *Shades of a Blue Orphanage* in spring 1972, again attracted cult status but did not sell as well as was merited. Frank from Decca tells how its seeming lack of commercial potential raised a question mark over whether they should be re-signed. It is humbling to hear that the company's head of promotion cited the support I gave their music as the reason for choosing to persist with the relationship.

Late 1972 saw the release of the single 'Whiskey in the Jar', delivering record sales success at last with this Lynott-arranged interpretation of a traditional Irish song of a highwayman being betrayed by his lover. Although Phil had always claimed he did not seek to be part of a singles band, he was to recognise the benefits of 'Whiskey in the Jar's success, not least the many appearances on *Top of The Pops* where he enjoyed being in attractive company. His own track 'Yellow Pearl' was adopted as its theme music in 1982.

I performed on their third album, *Vagabonds of the Western World*, on a track called 'The Hero and the Madman', albeit confined to a speaking part. Being all-too-familiar with Phil's fast-living lifestyle, it was fascinating to see the other side of him, focusing on his work in the studio, utterly in pursuit of perfection. I was reminded recently that I should have billed for the voiceover work, although the invoice may now seem a little tardy.

The Hero, rode a white horse
Across the desert
To where his woman was
He'd been riding
For four days
When he saw the tower...

As I think back to our encounters over the years, some pictures remain vivid in my mind. The café on the Place d'Armes in Luxembourg, where Phil slid his bass guitar out its case and practised al fresco as we sat outside and drank coffee. He was always compelling company.

Our relationship remained close, and I was so sad that he succumbed to temptation. Although he covered the effects of his excesses well for many years, keeping his challenges from those who could help him most, the long-term impact was starting to become clear.

After our paths had not crossed for a couple of years, Phil appeared alongside Slade towards the end of 1985 on a Tyne Tees TV show I was hosting called *Razzmatazz*, performing his solo track called '19' with Roger George and Brian Downey. Afterwards, Phil, Noddy Holder and I caught up and spent time reminiscing about the gigs at the Rainbow in London where I had introduced Thin Lizzy on stage as Slade's support act, and the band had performed in what was a regular pairing with Suzi Quatro.

Back in departures at Newcastle airport, Phil and I grabbed a snack and the conversation edged into the sort of honesty friends can have. He was having problems with his career, his family and his health. Although he looked in reasonable shape, his voice told a different story with the characteristic nasal sound often associated with the snorting of recreational drugs. The story was a familiar one: at his level, what the star wants the star gets, no matter how unwise.

I told him how much people loved him and wanted the best for him. Phil reassured me – and himself – that his issues were now in the past, and vowed he had resolved to be cleaner. He spoke of his hopes for his music and family, sliding open his briefcase to show me the Christmas cards he had written for his two daughters, and telling me of his plans to spend the festive season with them.

Over Christmas, he collapsed. Days later, less than a month after our final heart-to-heart, I was on-air when the announcement came through that my charismatic friend had died, aged just 36. I was devastated.

I had introduced him as a new act on Radio Luxembourg, and I had introduced his final TV performance. I have very fond memories of a hugely-talented performer and friend, whose career I happen to have bookended. He was a special guy.

8

ANOTHER DIMENSION

When you are aged 18 and your radio station boss asks for a volunteer, you put your hand up.

Radio Luxembourg's programme director Tony McArthur was excited about what had been unfolding in the US, where KSAN's general manager Tom Donahue was trying out new ideas on his FM station in San Francisco by playing free-form album tracks. Tom was an opinionated trend-setter, renowned for his article in *Rolling Stone* titled:'AM Radio is Dead and its Rotting Corpse is Stinking up the Airwaves'. Tony was keen to launch an adventurous programme on 208 which would be more exploratory, progressive and album-oriented. No-one else was doing it, and it was certainly unusual for even Radio Luxembourg to shift their turntables down a gear into $33\frac{1}{3}$ rpm.

Many presenters might be moved to militancy about being shunted away from the peak audience hours; for me, the proposed midnight show was absolutely the right opportunity. As a kid, I had loved the intimacy of radio late at night, with its more dedicated and discerning, audience. And, away from peak time, it afforded the chance for much more freedom.

My slot evolved from simply being titled *Kid Jensen* to *Another Dimension*, eventually settling on *Jensen's Dimensions*. Broadcast from midnight or one o'clock and ending at three in the morning, it was a good time to be on-air. Competition for late night ears was certainly limited, with BBC Radio 1 and 2 holding hands for *Night Ride*, promising 'Swinging sounds on and off the record' before closing the curtains at Broadcasting House completely at two o'clock.

The music I played excited me, and I devoured all the music mags from *Record Mirror* to *Melody Maker* and *Rolling Stone* to keep abreast of the latest insight. Back then, when a band changed record label, it was much like the hot news of a football transfer. I wanted to platform the bands and albums that were being written about, and truly embrace the music of the moment. As a listener you know when you are being conned and fooled; so, as a presenter you must be authentic.

The programme settled into a relaxed, almost hippie-flavoured presentation sound with a slower, quieter approach than the frantic earlier evening hours of Luxembourg's pop programmes. In recognition of the likely factions tuned-in, I even adopted a suitably kaftan-and-beads sign off at the end of each programme: 'Goodbye and good love', a phrase I puzzlingly sustained for some years.

The newspapers referred to me as playing 'Hard rock', but the late-night fare was so much more than that. This was a remarkable era for music, from the Sex Pistols to Joni Mitchell, and the format of *Dimensions* was just the right approach at the right time to attract attention from listeners, record labels and artists. The power of Radio Luxembourg meant it was rarely a struggle to persuade the biggest names to make the journey to see us. Joni was always a pleasure to talk to, opening up with such honesty and good humour, taking herself less seriously that her lyrics might suggest.

A midnight bang on the huge iron-clad door echoed around the château as I prepared to go on-air one night in 1971. Opening it cautiously, we found an exhausted Peter Gabriel and Phil Collins on the doorstep, clutching a copy of their album *Nursery Cryme,* the first to feature Phil Collins on drums and its striking Paul Whitehead cover depicting a Victorian croquet game with severed skulls lying on the lawn. Keen to gain exposure, they had hopped in their compact car and headed from London to the Ardennes Mountains, bound for the Grand Duchy. Four hundred miles later, the third Genesis album was safely on the turntable being heard by millions for the first time.

Alice Cooper visited too a couple of times, prompting an invitation from him to catch up subsequently. New York was the setting for our second encounter during dress rehearsals for his 'shock rock' US tour, his dress being the typical zips, black T-shirt and hair dangling down two feet longer than anyone else's. Over drinks and food in the Bowery, New York's oldest thoroughfare, I was shown one of the dark theatrics for the climax of the show: a frighteningly realistic guillotine designed by the Amazing Randi, then a magician and escape artist, but in later life a professional sceptic. That evening, the guillotine was tested out ahead of being used on stage. I declined to participate. Alice was to discover golf to escape from the world he had created around himself, and it was clear to see why.

Lengthy tracks dominated the *Dimensions* programme, and music was segued together in a way rarely heard at the time on UK radio, where presenters habitually talked in and out of every song in the time-honoured *Family Favourites* way. It always made me smile when the lovely David Hamilton used to deliver the big build up to his on-air afternoon 'tea break' on Radio 1, the one occasion when he dared to play a couple of songs in a row.

The stature of the station and the regard artists seemed to have for the programme was becoming clear. Jim Morrison from the Doors approached me at one Isle of Wight Festival. 'Luxembourg is just a massive station,' he remarked as we grabbed a drink. 'And you're always on it,' I replied.

I am also still amused by the ad for the Pop Proms at the Royal Albert Hall, which headlined with my name and John Peel's, with 'Led Zeppelin' printed in small font beneath. Years later, I was flattered to be asked to introduce Led Zeppelin's final show at Earls Court in London. As I stepped on stage, the band's legendary manager Peter Grant presented me with an engraved silver goblet in recognition of my support. For the lad who dreamed of being part of bands and the music scene, this was the closest I ever got.

Before his days with the Eagles, Joe Walsh came over from Cleveland, Ohio with his bandmates from the James Gang. A regular listener to Radio Luxembourg on short wave, he asked for a QSL card, which was one of the special cards radio buffs collected to authenticate their radio listening to stations from afar. We keep in touch to this day, and Joe still talks about that meeting and his fondness for the station.

Wishbone Ash impressed me from our earliest meetings in the early Seventies. With their unusual line-up of two lead guitars, rhythm and bass, plus an excellent drummer, they mastered a sort of pseudo-jazz, a very musical rock sound, creating some timeless songs. Paul Gambaccini was also captivated by the band. At the time of their debut he worked as a young writer for *Rolling Stone* magazine, an influential publication which was hipper than hip, with its writers themselves almost emerging as stars. Paul came over to Luxembourg to talk to me about the band at their recommendation, starting a friendship with him which was to last a lifetime.

Santana were a class act, introduced to me by one of my flatmates, Lloyd Mayes, a professional basketball player from Washington DC. At the time, the band's new album was an impressive mellow jazz and blues offering and Lloyd suggested I air it on *Jensen's Dimensions*. As Carlos Santana and his crew had evidently been in a spacey, chilled-out mood when assembling the album, I thought that I should listen in darkness to create the right mood in the studio. That blackout was an error of judgement, as witnessed by listeners when they heard the track fade and the record hit the runout groove. Some troubled to call in, worried I had been kidnapped or befallen some other fate, until the night watchman was alerted to wake me up.

As *Jensen's Dimensions* came to a close in the early hours of each morning, I said my listener goodbyes and then emerged into Luxembourg's night air, with nowhere to drink and unwind given the city's unsympathetic licensing hours. Solutions were inventive, including the discreet venue accessible only by scaling five floors up a fire escape. We then clambered across the roof in the dim light of the night, opened an unmarked yellow door and climbed back down into what was a drinking den full of familiar faces, many speaking English. The police, the Gendarmerie, also appeared to spend a lot of time there for reasons other than investigation into after-hours drinking.

Luxy presenters were booked frequently to perform at Blow Up Club, which was so intimate you would turn around at the bar and end up almost on stage. After our sets, the floor would be swiftly cleared, allowing bands to drag their equipment into place, with the organisers trusting my instinct on which new live acts might be well-received by the crowd of twenty and thirty-somethings. As I mull over the roster now, I shiver when I think of how many of the recordings of those priceless early performances from rock's huge names have now vanished.

By 1973, I had heard about a new band called Queen, described by *Rolling Stone* magazine as a 'funky, energetic English quartet'. I loved their energy; but knew that Radio 1 might be a little more suspicious about airplay, given their music was loud and they had pesky long hair. Having performed in Germany at their first overseas gig, they were booked at the Blow Up before returning to the UK. I found them incredible guys with a great attitude, and I liked them as people: Roger, the incredible drummer; Brian, the gifted guitarist; John, the quiet bass player; and Freddie, the showman. Although I would love a chance to listen back to that gig now, I remember quietly thinking, at that earliest stage of their career, there was something just a little too derivative about that night's performance.

After the gig we adjourned to the Holiday Inn, Freddie theatrical rather than camp, holding court and telling stories to his harem. They were not just tales of sex, drugs and rock and roll, there was an air of intellectualism in their conversation. These are truly unique memories of a time and place in music history.

Rick Wakeman from Yes made an impact at the Blow Up when he visited as part of the promotion for *Six Wives of Henry VIII,* the solo album inspired by a book he saw on an airport bookstall. A chest freezer was pushed on stage – from which he emerged. By contrast, Rick's first impression of me, when our paths crossed just after an interview by Stuart Henry, was that I looked like an angelic choir boy from the local church. His stage appearances have always impressed, being such an imposing big guy, yet delivering beautiful melodies which stretched the imaginations of the audience.

Radio Luxemborug's Villa Louvigny boasted its own magnificent concert hall, built in 1952 for the RTL Orchestra. In 1972 it hosted the Beach Boys, and the impeccable harmonies from *Pet Sounds* echoed off the walls of a venue more typically known for its classical performance. Mike Love, Dennis Wilson, Carl Wilson, Ricky Fataar, Blondie Chaplin and Al Jardine played with a backing band featuring Captain and Tennille.

In May 1972 the Grateful Dead performed there, a band I believed had changed the course of contemporary music in their seven years of existence. We planned to beam out their set on short wave around the world, on three FM stations in Germany, on long wave in France and on the famous 208 metres wavelength. In a departure from the usual approach, the transmitters were set to burn all night to broadcast the whole three-hour set live.

The band was particularly huge in France, so interest was high when we announced the gig. It grew further when one of the French announcers made the error of implying on-air – to the whole of Europe – that it was free to attend, as opposed to the band having not been paid. Consequently, we were besieged with huge numbers of people arriving by train or plane into Luxembourg desperate to see their heroes, far more than could be accommodated. The baying crowd could be heard outside, and the Villa's moat came in useful in a scene which came to appear worrying like the Storming of the Bastille.

As the band tuned up, I was asked to pass on a note to the bass player Phil Lesh. Walking on stage to hand it over, one of the Hell's Angels roadies confronted me. The malevolent expression on his face indicated my presence was more than unwelcome, and his words were unrepeatable. Hearing a click, I looked down to see a switchblade knife in my stomach. Jerry Garcia, the Grateful Dead's guitarist and vocalist, came to the rescue, calling out 'It's OK, he's with us.' My disappointed potential assailant wandered off in search of someone else to annoy. Although tempted to report the incident, I concluded his entourage looked like one I would best not get on bad terms with.

Pulse racing, I introduced the band, forsaking my lengthy planned citation of the band's colourful heritage for little more than 'Ladies and gentlemen – the Grateful Dead.' I just wanted to escape. Drama aside, the Hell's Angels outfit appeared to enjoy their appearance in Luxembourg and even extended their stay in the city afterwards just to see our mighty transmitters for themselves.

○

When Mick Jagger suggests he would like you to join him on the tour plane as the Stones dashed around the United States, you do not argue. This was the band's private tour plane, with their iconic red tongue and lips logo emblazoned on the tail fin. It was winter 1972, and they were promoting the album *Exile on*

Main Street. My presence with the band en route was not wholly popular, with American record producer Marshall Chess, the record label manager, making clear I was not welcome. I know that because the seating arrangements on the small aircraft meant I witnessed every heated word.

On touchdown in Philadelphia a police escort and outriders accompanied us as we sped through the streets to the Spectrum, a huge ice hockey venue which had gained a reputation as the home of the biggest rock names. When I asked Bill Wyman where I might sit to watch, he generously handed me an Access All Areas pass and gestured to the stage: 'Sit with us.' I did – witnessing a performance from the greats from a vantage point just feet behind them. On occasions now, I catch vintage footage of the gig with the camera panning round to catch my young face sandwiched between Mick and Bill.

After the concert it was onwards to Pittsburgh, from where take-off was subsequently delayed. Given this was a private plane, airport procedures were a little less formal and we disembarked for the wait. Killing time, one of the guys got out a football and the band invited me to join in a kickabout on the runway. A career in radio offers many surreal experiences, but little compares to playing football with the Rolling Stones at midnight at a Pittsburgh airport.

9

GOT TO BE THERE

It was Christmas Eve, 1974.

A flight attendant for the Icelandic airline Loftleiðir called Guðrún was reluctantly staying for a few nights in Luxembourg on standby over the festive season. She was deeply missing her home in Iceland, a country which traditionally made such an occasion of Christmas. Back then, Loftleiðir, later called Icelandair, was the cheapest way to cross the Atlantic; the forerunner of the Freddie Laker routes which pushed forward the 'low cost – no-frills' airline business model used subsequently by millions of passengers.

Guðrún was planning to study at university, but had taken a year out to work with the airline, as it seemed a glamorous job and an opportunity to see the world. International journeys in that era had a real sense of occasion; pilots were not simply regarded as bus drivers, and all staff were offered attractive perks.

As a single guy, too far away from Vancouver to travel home, I had volunteered to stay in Luxembourg to cover the seasonal shifts on the station, allowing the English guys a chance to make their short journeys home. My Christmas Eve mid-evening show ended and I walked out into the cold December air into a quiet city. The Duchy took its religious holidays seriously and its people had left town and returned to their family homes.

The Black Bess was empty when I dropped in, so cheery conversation was initiated with the club manager in the absence of anyone else with whom to make merry. Our chat was then interrupted by a lively party bursting in, fresh from a long dinner. One of them was Guðrún.

Doing his best to liven up the night, my flatmate Golly jumped on duty and devised an impromptu competition on stage. Contestants were instructed to blow up balloons, with the inflator of the largest one winning. There was no doubt that Guðrún had seized victory, until one of her crowd – an annoying pilot – burst her bulging balloon with his cigar. As she had merely missed out on winning a copy of *The Best of Judge Dread*, which I rightly guessed was not to her taste, I whispered in her ear that I could offer much better prizes.

Guðrún had dark hair combed-back, lovely eyes and a bubbly personality which reacted to everyone around her. Brilliant with people, always remembering names and personal details, I could see why she was doing the job she was. Guðrún was simply great to be with.

She tells me now she thought I was Icelandic on first sight, given my looks and hair, and that is what charmed her. She had no idea I was on the radio, and preferred classical and ballet to rock and pop.

As we chatted, I felt the sort of immediate spark you experience rarely in life, and a hunger to see her again. Luckily, my colleague Tony Prince had invited me to a party on Christmas Day, so on the spur of the moment I invited her to join me. As we parted from the Black Bess and went our separate ways, I assured her I would be in touch to let her know the arrangements for our rendezvous.

Messaging in the era before mobile phones was a complex affair. Star-crossed lovers would arrange to meet at local landmarks at agreed times, and one imagines many promising relationships were thwarted by a change in plans or a tardy bus arrival which could not be communicated. It very nearly happened to us. As Guðrún was staying in a hotel, I resorted to leaving messages on the switchboard number, messages she failed to receive. She tells me she still remembers how crestfallen she was, and how she gave up and went out with her friends instead to try to make something of the festive night. It was only on her return to her accommodation as Christmas Eve turned into Christmas Day that she received my message, explaining that I had discovered Tony's social event was a sit-down meal and that I had not felt able to take along a guest without an invitation. Apologies accepted, we agreed to attend a Boxing Day party together instead.

The relationship quickly blossomed, even though Guðrún's travels around the world meant our time together was sparse. In those days, even talking on the phone was a major event. Making an international call required advance booking so that the operators around the world could be poised to plug in the correct wires to unite the nations. Relief came when she confided about her Luxembourg love to one of her aunties, who volunteered that any future calls could be booked to her phone, affording Guðrún some certainty and privacy.

Guðrún listened to my voice on the radio whenever she could, even driving in the darkness to the south coast of Iceland just to reach the point on raised land where the Radio Luxembourg signal could be heard beaming across the sea. When the lyrics of Clifford T Ward's 'Home Thoughts From Abroad' crackled through, she knew it was played for her: 'I miss you, I really do.' To this day, his haunting vocals take my mind back instantly to those colourful Grand Duchy days. Such is love.

'How do you say, 'Will you marry me' in Icelandic?' I asked Guðrún just two months after our first encounter. She told me. Next day, on the strength of her proposal, I phoned and we arranged to choose the ring.

After toasting with Möet champagne and nibbling on smoked salmon in my apartment to celebrate our engagement, we slid out for a romantic dinner. Although we had only met up a few times before the proposal, our partnership simply seemed right. I can conclude no other than a guardian angel on my shoulder had led me in the direction of choosing my wife and lifetime soul mate.

We were married in June, journeying back to Guðrún's home to exchange vows in Dómkirkjan í Reykjavík, the modest 18th century Reykjavík Cathedral where each session of the Icelandic parliament Alþingi begins with a Mass. Our partnership has now lasted over forty-five years, and she has been with me through all the ups and downs of my radio career.

Radio is never a nine-to-five job, particularly if your programmes do not even start until midnight. Aside from the commitments on-air, there are a host of other places you are required to be and people you must meet. It is also a world where social life and professional life dovetail, so on many occasions where I have had the privilege of rubbing shoulders some of music's top names, Guðrún has been by my side.

Given she hailed from another country and our musical heritage was so different, she was not always au fait with the top names with whom I was associating. Whilst most people were in awe of some of the accomplished, temperamental characters in the music world, Guðrún simply took them as she found them and was always true to herself. Mark Knopfler from Dire Straits may recall her innocently asking him what he did for a living. I do not know of any career advice she might have volunteered when he told her he was in dire straits.

○

The moonwalk is a dance move which will forever be associated with Michael Jackson. Known until 1983 as the backslide, with the dancer gliding backwards whilst their body actions suggest a forward motion, Michael's interpretation was to re-define the move. Its first public performance in March 1983 in front of a live audience at the Pasadena Civic Auditorium was witnessed by huge TV audiences two months later as part of the TV special, *Motown 25: Yesterday, Today, Forever.*

During his UK visit that year, he invited about half a dozen of us to a select get-together at a hotel on Park Lane. It is the sort of invitation you do not turn down and I went along with Guðrún. The wine and conversation flowed and it became one of those accidental nights it was good to part of. We smile to this day when we think back to the most memorable part of the evening – the moment when I turned around to witness Michael teaching Guðrún to do the moonwalk on the thick shag pile carpet.

His brother Jermaine had appeared on my programme as a guest the previous week, so I was fascinated when, later at that party, Michael came across purposefully, sat next to me and quietly asked: 'Did you speak to Jermaine? What did he say about me?' I told him truthfully that I could not recall the exact words, but that the comments were complimentary and not critical in any way. He listened carefully to my reassurance, just saying 'That's nice,' before walking away. Looking back, that worried enquiry gave something of an insight into his complex and insecure character.

I gather there has been a recent study of all the interviews from his high-profile period, and it appeared he was interviewed by me more than by anyone else. I always found him charming and friendly in person whilst, professionally, he was taking the mantle from Fred Astaire as the world's greatest song-and-dance man.

Michael and I had met earlier in summer 1979 during my time at Radio 1, when he guested on the *Roundtable* programme, where personalities were invited to review new tracks, a little like the Sixties TV show *Juke Box Jury*, with artists judging the work of their peers in the industry. He was on the interview circuit promoting *Off the Wall*. Remarkably, also booked that day was the quiet Beatle, George Harrison, eager for exposure for his eponymous new album. It is tragic that both those huge musical talents are now no longer with us.

When two artists of that calibre with mutual respect get together and feel at home in each other's company, a compelling programme is assured. We discussed singles by the Blues Brothers, Foreigner and Nicolette Larson, alongside the distinguished guests' own music. Michael was relaxed and on good form, creating an excellent vibe in the studio, where George felt at ease too. Michael opened-up about how challenging it had been to begin to write and then record his own songs, and asked George whether the Beatles had composed their own material right from their beginning. When George confirmed that was the case, Michael was incredulous: 'How did you ever manage that?' 'I don't know,' George retorted. 'They were clever little fellows.'

I took my lead from the artists when they appeared on *Roundtable*. Some were already familiar with the songs being discussed and just wanted to chat casually off-air as they played, while others put on their headphones, concentrated on the music and prepared a considered academic review of what they had heard. Michael and George took the listening seriously in their own ways, just as Elton did when on the programme, always keener to talk about others' music than their own. On this night, Michael was like a little kid, eager to hear the next song, George a little more laid-back.

Some years later I was invited to be part of an obituary for Michael, recorded some years before his death. Major broadcasters routinely prepare these tribute programmes well in advance for even the healthiest of key figures, and those invited to contribute duly adopt a fitting sorrowful tone as their words are recorded, even though the subject is probably at home at the time enjoying a bottle of wine. No-one taking part in the Jackson edition anticipated their words would be aired quite so soon afterwards.

10

GETTING KNOWN

Muriel Young was a legend. A beautiful sparkling actress and TV presenter/producer with a mischievous smile. She was also the in-vision announcer on the opening night of Associated-Rediffusion TV in London in 1955. She had recorded shows for Radio Luxembourg in the early Sixties, including the EMI show *Friday Spectacular* with Shaw 'Keep 'em peeled' Taylor.

It was through Muriel, by that time a director/producer at Granada, that I secured my first television opportunity when she invited me onto a talent show hosted by Dana, the Irish 1970 Eurovision Song Contest winner. The atmosphere and ethos of a TV studio was foreign to me at the time, as not only had I not done such work before, I had barely even watched TV in Luxembourg. None of us, apart from Paul Burnett, even possessed a TV set, which was perhaps one of the reasons why we all indulged in such a lively nightlife.

In spring 1974, Muriel appointed me to host a talent show called *Rock on with 45*, later just *45*. Reflecting on the programme in a Radio Luxembourg documentary which I only heard recently, Muriel was kind enough to say that, apart from the music, my contribution helped its success: 'He knows what he's talking about and he doesn't waste anybody's time, he just tells them what it is – and he speaks with such authority.'[9]

All the big names of the day guested on *45*, which was recorded

---

9   'This Is How It All Began': Radio Luxembourg documentary, 1974.

by Granada in Manchester and broadcast originally just to the north, but later nationally. I have a vague recollection of ABBA appearing on the 1974 Christmas show, although like so many precious performances I can sadly track down no record of the event. I am told they performed 'So Long', the first single from their eponymous third album. The group's artistry was always thoroughly impressive, with glowing production ideas and huge innovation.

On the journeys north to record the programme, we travelled alongside the likes of Bowie and Bolan in one of those wonderful old, seemingly spacious British Rail slam-door trains, creating a real sense on-board of togetherness from artists and production staff alike. The Bay City Rollers joined us on one occasion, whom I found nice guys. But it was my colleague Peter Powell who was most closely aligned with them on Radio Luxembourg, even adopting their tartan look to embrace Rollermania.

TV was a powerful vehicle, particularly with the colossal audiences each of the three channels commanded back then. The mighty *Coronation Street* was made by Granada too, and members of the soap's cast frequently eavesdropped on the recording of *45*. Grasping the stature of the show in the UK, but not yet knowing too well the difference between character and actor, I once greeted Pat Phoenix with a cheery 'Hello, Elsie.' She recognised me, and seemed nonplussed about the name I had chosen to use.

Our faces were often seen too in *Fabulous 208*, a best-selling pin-up magazine catering for teen pop music fans. Alongside *Jackie,* we knew it was big amongst our audience. Teenagers eagerly awaited the delivery of the latest edition so they might tear out their favourite moody faces to stick lovingly on their bedroom walls. The month I began at Luxembourg, your shilling would have bought an issue featuring Steve Marriott, Status Quo, Peter Noone from Herman's Hermits and a pin-up of young *Oliver!* actor Jack Wild. Given it was a true colourful burst of teenage music, fashion and beauty, the photographs of the Radio Luxembourg presenters had to complement the other glossy shots. The magazine's photographer used to come over to see us and help us strike a series of wacky poses, a little like the Monkees' stunts of a few years before.

Although I failed to grace the front cover of the January 1970 edition of *Fabulous 208*, the splash headline did promise a 'king-size colour' picture of me inside. By February 1970 I had clearly moved up a league, as the front page boasted 'Romantic Men in Colour', with me featured inside, wearing a leather jacket and vivid turquoise shirt, pictured alongside the familiar faces of the great George Best, actor Richard Beckinsale and Alan Osmond, the eldest of the Osmonds.

Listeners started to put a face to my name, and each time I returned to the UK I attracted those second glances from people who felt they knew me… from somewhere. Glam Rock fans gathered by the Granada gate waiting for the artists – and me – to emerge. Whilst I hope I never became a show-off, I was glad to be invited to parties and become part of the great tradition of the entertainment business. I found it flattering to be greeted in the streets. People were generally friendly, and I always tried to reciprocate. Like a politician, you are only successful if people like you.

Advertisers too were keen to draw on our equity and influence, particularly with younger generations. They paid the station to seed their commercial brands in the natural flow of the presenter's on-air dialogue with their audience. Rather than pause for a thirty-second ad spot, we were instructed to enthuse about a product personally, in the way that did not become legal on UK-based radio until almost forty years afterwards. This seeming endorsement was a powerful device for a station facing commercial competition from an ever-more powerful ITV, with its growing audience and stature with advertisers.

One memorable Radio Luxembourg client was the Tea Council, which seemed to have the ambition of turning the comforting lukewarm drink into a vibrant contemporary hero, thanks to radio advertising leaning on the image and reputation of Radio Luxembourg. The budget for the campaign was significant, so, for an odd period on-air, when we were not talking about music we were contriving links about tea: 'I'm feeling a little tired right now, I think I'll have a cup of tea whilst we listen to… the Beatles.' 'That song's a great pick-me-up, and Tony has just brought me a nice pick-me-up – a delicious steaming cup of tea.' Had the advertiser been a specific tea brand, listeners would have grasped the arrangement, but as it was more generic our audience seemed increasingly puzzled by our obsession, prompting one American in Germany to write to say how clever he thought we were in using the term 'tea bags' to disguise our references to drugs.

After the success of our English service, our French service colleagues at RTL were experimenting with the Radio Luxembourg programme style on their transmitters and I was selected to host the bilingual show, owing to my Canadian background. In the west of Canada, French lessons were compulsory for five years of secondary education as French is one of the country's two official languages, and the mother tongue of a fifth of the population.

The French service enjoyed popularity in Paris for the same reasons the English service was an attractive choice for UK listeners. It was a privilege to be invited to broadcast, initially from their Paris studios from where Rosko had amassed a huge following as 'le Président Rosko'. Unlike the English service, the French offering had been allowed to broadcast live programmes from their destination country, sending them back via landline direct to the powerful transmitters in Luxembourg.

On the days I was required, an obliging friend collected me after my *Dimensions* programme at night and drove the four hours to the centre of Paris, delivering me just as the sun rose over the Eiffel Tower and another day began. It was as poetic as it sounds. My shows from the studios on the rue Bayard included a smattering of basic French and an increasing amount of English, possibly a reason why the project was short-lived.

Familiar faces are always a welcome sight when you are thousands of miles away from home. On one occasion, in a restaurant in Luxembourg, I was tapped on the shoulder. Turning round, I was delighted to see Christine, the smiley girl I had left behind back home in Canada when I left so abruptly, and the one who had prompted the premature end to my schooldays.

Rarely was I homesick, but I did feel a pang when my parents were splitting up, and I made the decision to return to Canada. Press interviews from the time also quote me as saying that I was uneasy at the time with my programmes on Luxembourg: 'I didn't want to play what somebody else told me to play, I wanted to play my own thing. I thought that I could best put across my own personality by playing the music I enjoy playing.' I have now little recollection of any of those musical anxieties, which clearly meant so much at the time.

By then, my family had moved to Whitehorse, the capital of northwest Canada's Yukon territory, which was very different from Vancouver, not least the sub-Arctic weather with bitterly cold winters but twenty hours of sun on summer days. Their next-door neighbours kept a wolf in the pen next to us, in this spirited community who referred ominously to 'going outside' when they ventured any further than a ten-mile radius of their town. With wild animals on your route when you did so, it all seemed a long way from Carnaby Street.

CKRW was the local station, with an MOR format and a transmission footprint extending farther north and farther west than any other Canadian radio operation. Although I hosted some programmes, I soon realised my future was not to be there, or in Whitehorse generally, so I was emboldened by a telegram from

Radio Luxembourg's programme director who asked whether I fancied returning for my own regular show.

From newspaper cuttings I have only seen recently, I gather I was being missed by listeners who apparently petitioned for my return. One publicity photograph shows me on the steps of 10 Downing Street for reasons which escape me. Another animated shot from the time depicts my return. Dodging the London traffic, I am pictured outside the Swiss Centre at Leicester Square, arms outstretched, beneath the huge news tickertape display bearing the message 'Kid Jensen returns to 208'. The picture was published centre-spread in *Fabulous 208* magazine, accompanied by touching comment from colleagues 'telexed from Luxembourg': 'It just ain't been the same without you. Welcome back to where you belong, Kid. Your old mate, Paul Burnett.' Typically, Bob Stewart took a different angle: 'Hello kiddo, I told you six months, and you'd want to come home. You're two months early.'

These were heady days, and such is our changed media world it is difficult to imagine a late-night radio presenter now receiving such a fanfare on the strength of returning to a radio station.

By 1975, after five years back on-air in Luxembourg accompanied by more TV appearances, my UK profile had grown and I became hopeful of a new opportunity. Maybe it was frustration about Radio Luxembourg's wobbly signal compared with the clear FM signals beaming out from the UK's new commercial stations, or the crazy working hours, but more likely it was because I had fallen in love and wanted to plan a life together with Guðrún.

The BBC's Doreen Davies paid a timely visit to Luxembourg with her husband Derek Mills, both leading lights at Radio 1 and Radio 2 with a key role in the Corporation's hiring and firing. Doreen was a determined operator with a real love for the glam and glitter of pop. She smoked, drank lots of coffee and always wore a huge trademark rosette of flowers. A remarkable character, for whom I and many of her radio generation have respect and affection, Doreen died in the summer of 2020.

Whilst in the Grand Duchy to attend a conference, Doreen visited Radio Luxembourg and was shown by the commissionaire into the presenters' 'playpen', where we presenters hung out when not on-air. Doreen sidled over and whispered in my ear, enquiring discreetly whether I had any desire to move to Radio 1. This was exactly the news I had hoped for – a chance to broadcast to the UK on my dream radio station and live in London. Seeing my face light up, she then cautioned that I might find relating fully to the station's audience a challenge, as I had yet to experience the nuances of British life. Doreen suggested I acclimatise myself by spending some time working at one of the local commercial stations then opening in the UK. Luckily, when interviewed I had always welcomed the arrival of new commercial radio competition, suggesting that if the status quo were never challenged there was a risk of stagnation: 'You wonder if everyone's listening to you because there is nothing else on the radio.'[10]

To walk out on my huge international Radio Luxembourg audience in favour of a small local station in a new country was a gamble, but I considered the ultimate prize of a place at BBC Radio 1 worth the risk.

Doreen's advice to dunk myself in British culture was promptly taken and I broke the news to the stoic Luxy management, who had become accustomed to presenters treading the well-worn path to Radio 1. After seven-and-a-half years, I prepared to wave farewell to the patch of Europe where I had spent a formative chunk of my life – an experience which had been all I had dreamed of and more.

---

10 *Deejay*, November 1972.

11.
A BRITISH APPRENTICESHIP

'Radio in jeans' was the label attached by the broadcasting regulator to the scattering of new UK commercial radio stations in the Seventies. After fifty years of BBC monopoly, listeners were being treated to an additional, more casual offering, struggling on-air at a challenging economic time for the country under the new Conservative Government. London was the home for the first two launches: the news station LBC and the 'general entertainment station' Capital, followed by others dotted around the UK. Any thought of national commercial radio was seen as thoroughly far-fetched.

Dennis Maitland was a key early mover in the new wave of stations. I knew him from his role as director of sales at Radio Luxembourg, a grown-up based in the London offices rather than one of the Luxembourg-based pranksters. If I was a disc jockey, he was very much a desk jockey. Pinstripe-suited with a healthy head of hair and a bushy moustache, he was worldly-wise and gifted in client dealings, with a dry sense of humour and the determination to deliver. Before his spell with Radio Luxembourg he had been the administration director for the successful and most professional of the offshore pirate stations, Radio London. Upon the promise of UK commercial radio, Dennis joined the consortium which successfully won the franchise in 1974 for the Nottingham area. Then the sole commercial station in the East Midlands, it served a potential audience of around a million people.

Taking Doreen's advice to identify a suitable home for my British probation, I leaned on Dennis. As managing director of his new Radio Trent 301, he offered me a contract to become part of its launch presentation team. I suspect he thought a recognised radio name from Radio Luxembourg would prove an asset, to complement the other presenters who had been hired. Although most of them also had relevant experience, they were less likely to be familiar to listeners as they had simply not yet been heard on-air in the area.

Billboard magazine from March 1975 reported my appointment: 'Kid Jensen is leaving Radio Luxembourg to join Radio Trent, the Nottingham commercial station, but will continue with discotheque and television work.'

Guðrún gave up her work at the airline to join me in the UK, and just a couple of weeks before the station began broadcasting, we arrived in Nottingham. It was a city I grew to like quickly, with fine pubs and decent music venues. Having found a house in Ruddington on the outskirts of the city, before moving to Radcliffe-on-Trent, we began living together full-time. Many married couples will relate to the early challenges of that adjustment. DIY was the source of our first row. Having had a father who knew what he was doing in that field, Guðrún had inherited those skills and believed she knew how to do everything. As did I.

Trent broadcast from premises in the heart of the city, opposite an 18th century pub called the Royal Children. On a warm July day in 1975, just a month after the first Common Market referendum and on the eve of my 25th birthday, we prepared to go on-air, with a pioneering team of just over fifty people dedicated to the cause, ready to broadcast eighteen hours each day.

On Day One I hosted the afternoon show, preceding a half-hour evening news programme followed by a phone-in to meet the 'meaningful speech' obligations then placed on the early commercial stations. In the station's promotional material, Trent was keen to make abundantly clear that I would be playing a 'very different style of music' from my Luxembourg days, promising 'more melodious music, plus news items, sports reports, traffic news and what's on and where to go.'

This local talk element was new to me in a sense, although I had worked on some small stations back home. Luxembourg had attracted a huge international audience, whilst Trent focused just on Nottinghamshire. Although very much a music radio station, it was much more community-based, not talking at people, instead a hallmark of a warmer, friendlier, more sincere sound. I was happy to integrate local information in the show, reading out local diary items and delivering remotes from such places as the annual Newark and Notts Agricultural Show.

Smartly-dressed, sitting in the studio wearing a white jacket and vibrant shirt, I spoke earnestly in a launch day interview aired on ATV about how 'invigorated' I was by Trent's local credentials: 'Luxembourg was a terrific experience, with the accent more on records and the selling of records, which is an important source of revenue for 208. Here, of course the community comes first.'

A small local newspaper in the city, *Nottingham Voice*, reported generously on my arrival: 'Trent have scooped a big-name disc jockey in Kid Jensen, who in recent months has been hosting a rock music show on Radio Luxembourg and a young-at-heart pop show on Granada television.' The article concluded, however, with the sobering 'If you're under thirty you'll probably have heard his mid-Atlantic drawl before, but otherwise his name will mean nothing.'

Another key difference between Radio Luxembourg and Radio Trent was a keen sense of competition. When 208 came on-air at night-time, BBC Radio 1 was asleep; we were alone and ruled supreme. At Radio Trent, we saw the BBC – and its Radio Nottingham specifically – as a direct competitor. Very successful at the time and much-loved, the role it played in the community was highly-regarded. Whilst Trent did make some contribution to the area's pride, culture and business, its music format lent more of the Radio 1 or Luxembourg feel. As time has passed, I have developed great respect for the people who work in BBC local radio. That sort of public service radio might not be viewed as quite as glamorous as the music stations, but the companionship, informational value and emotional connection it delivers is impressive.

The charts of the time were replete with summery pop, with teen bands such as the Osmonds and Bay City Rollers fighting for primacy each week on the cover of *Jackie* magazine. Trent, however, had installed a relatively adult music policy at the outset. In my 1975 TV interview, I talked delicately about Trent being about 'popular music. But by that, I don't just mean simply the Top 20 but other things as well that our programme director feels would be suitable for our programming.'

For a music artist to build a reputation, radio remained the key route, given the colourful breakfast and daytime TV sofas had yet to arrive, and the online world had yet to be connected. As UK commercial radio was still a totally local operation, stars had to travel up and down the motorways just for a ten-minute interview, or diarise the time to call in when performing locally to address the stations' appreciable audiences.

David Cassidy journeyed to Trent in 1976 to promote his album *Home Is Where The Heart Is*. Carving out a successful career as a solo artist following his fame on TV's *The Partridge Family*, fans queued outside the station down Castle Gate to catch a glimpse of the New Jersey star with his long hair, tasselled jacket and ready smile. I remember him as being friendly, happy to meet people and to pose for photographs. Although it is easy to regard him just as a pin-up boy, he had substantial talent and I found his songs well-chosen and well-sung.

My afternoon show on Trent seemed to be well-received, and

by February the following year I was shifted up the schedule to the mid-morning show. With most presenters called upon to host six shows a week in commercial radio, I was also asked to present the Saturday afternoon programme, featuring football results delivered by wry moustachioed sports colleague Martin Johnson, at an exciting time for Nottingham Forest, then managed by the irrepressible Brian Clough.

At weekends, Trent's spacious building was deserted, with the commercial and management staff away with their families and only the on-air staff on-site. Getting motivated for weekend shows on most stations can be a challenge, with the hustle and bustle absent and the atmosphere dead.

On one of those quiet, yet beautifully warm mid-Seventies Saturday afternoons, I was preparing to go on-air, sitting on the first floor in front of the open window, with the sun shining through and no hint of a breeze. Suddenly, the old sash window slammed itself shut. No-one else had entered, and the sturdy yellow door to my left stayed closed. At the same time, another of the windows partially opened. The room was silent, and I looked around to see no-one. Then, another window behind me creaked and closed… and I joined the lengthy list of occupants of the building who had witnessed something odd. The ghostly sightings were perhaps to be expected from the radio station's characterful four-storey 18th century home, formerly a women's hospital, with its cool subterranean studios having once served as the morgue.

My spell at Trent was nearly not to be. The day before my debut programme in Nottingham, a call came from Capital Radio's programme controller Aidan Day, later immortalised in the 1977 Clash song 'Capital Radio' which attacked that station's mainstream music policy: 'Get the word from Aiden Day, He picks all the hits to play, To keep you in your place all day.' Capital had launched in London a couple of years previously, and Aiden was suddenly looking to fill the shoes of rock show presenter Nicky Horne for a period. With the ink already dry on my Trent contract, the timing for the call could not have been poorer, even though that initial agreement extended to a period of just three months.

Sadly, at that stage in my career I did not enjoy the benefit of a thick-skinned agent who might have been prepared to risk Trent's wrath by negotiating a last-minute switch for me to the much larger London station. One of the benefits of investing in the services of an agent is their role in such difficult conversations, and I engaged a number of them in later days. Sixties hitmaker Adam Faith, who had discovered Sandie Shaw and managed Leo Sayer, asked to represent me at one stage, although we did not reach an agreement. Other agents to whom I am grateful through the years include John Miles, Anthony Blackburn and Roger De Courcey, all bringing wise counsel, a bulging contact book and, in Roger's case, Nookie Bear.

My first agent almost steered me into a second career as a singer. The youthful energy of a bright young Londoner from Radio Luxembourg called David Collins more than made up for his relative lack of experience in the role. He delivered an offer from Warner Brothers for me to record the McCartney track 'Bluebird', as heard on the album *Band on the Run*. It's an excellent, timeless track, and there seemed a definite yet puzzling appetite for my vocals for a single. After much internal agony, and persistence from David, I turned down the flattering offer, concluding that singing was simply not territory where I felt at home.

Press headlines in the Seventies made depressing reading. It was the decade of strikes, power cuts and rubbish piled on the street. Industrial relations in the UK were at a low, and broadcasting was no exception, with Trent and LBC gaining a reputation for being particularly fraught. Towards the end of my time at Trent there was a serious fracture in relations between Dennis Maitland and his first programme director. The latter had been dismissed in May 1976, and the matter became heated when his union, the Association of Broadcasting and Allied Staffs (ABAS) supported his case. Fellow presenters bearing placards marched outside Trent's Georgian front door, picketing the premises, and a sit-in for a day-and-a-half ensued in one of the studios, with food smuggled in to sustain the protestors via the graveyard at the rear of the premises. As might be expected, the episode became a major news story locally as this brave new venture became part of a drama.

There was a personal complication. I was not a member of the union in dispute, and therefore had neither reason nor justification to strike. Without that defence, it seemed wrong to let Dennis Maitland down, not least following the faith he had shown in me. My work as a columnist, however, had led to my signing up to membership of a different union: The National Union of Journalists. I duly sought the view of its Father of the Chapel, the rather quaint name for the local co-ordinator, who advised clearly that the dispute should not involve me. I should add that the NUJ had its own separate dispute at Trent that year. Little wonder the station's industrial record caused furrowed brows at its regulator.

As a novel music-playing NUJ member, therefore, I was the only programme presenter who turned up for work, with the remainder of the schedule filled with tapes of continuous music. For a few difficult days, I arrived to face a walk of shame through pickets of angry staff to get into the building with tensions running high, cat-calling and hugely-unpleasant remarks from some of the team lined up outside. Inside, I found my letters ripped up or thrown out the window, and even threats to my dog. For me, doing my best in a new job and trying to make my way in a new country, I found the hot-headedness hugely upsetting. Radio was surely supposed to be about access and entertainment, not this.

The nasty experience was something I had never come across anywhere else in the world I had worked. Ruining relations with several colleagues, the incident leaves a sour taste in my mouth to this day.

Arriving home after my show ended one day, I took a welcome phone call from Derek Chinnery, who ran BBC Radio 1. He explained that Rosko was leaving the station to return to the US to be close to his Hollywood film producer father, who was ill in LA, and asked if I would replace him. Rosko – or Emperor Rosko – to give Mike Pasternak his full official on-air name, was the fast-talking, rasping American voice who famously, on the first day of Radio 1 in 1967, prompted newsreader John Dunn to begin his news bulletin within the *Midday Spin* lunchtime programme with the words: 'And now the news – in English.'

The Radio 1 contract on offer was just six months in length, but I gave no thought to the brevity, or anything else. With all the upset at Trent, this fantastic offer was perfectly timed. Not only did I want the opportunity in London, I would have ran down the motorway to get there.

This was like joining the Beatles.

12

PERFECT PITCH

Brian Clough was starting his journey to local hero status during my spell in Nottingham. Having walked through the gate at the City Ground in 1975, just months before I arrived at Radio Trent, in a short time he was to take Forest from thirteenth in the old Division Two to a league title and back-to-back European Cups.

The Clough reputation was unparalleled. One anecdote told of when a colleague walked into his office to find him listening to his favourite singer. 'Did you know,' Clough asked him, 'Sinatra met me once?'

My encounter with Old Big 'Ead came when I was invited back to Nottingham at the height of his success to support a Junior Reds presentation. Walking into the tunnel from the pitch, I caught sight of Brian at the far end sporting his trademark green sweatshirt, poised to lead his team out – in silence, in contrast to the noisy adversaries. I made my way through the tunnel to be introduced to him and held out my hand to shake his. He determinedly ignored the gesture, folding his arms across his chest as if in a wall about to face a free kick, and stared at me in a disarming way for some uncomfortable time before walking away without a word.

When introduced later that afternoon to Brian's son Nigel, who was also to become a well-known figure in the game, I remarked that I was glad at least one member of the family was talking to me. The Clough score grew as I was introduced to Brian's wonderful wife Barbara in the boardroom afterwards, as we joined the good and the great over steak and beans. Such was her charm I was prompted to wonder what I was missing about her husband's true character.

Ice hockey had been my game back home in Canada and its top players were my heroes so, on my arrival here, I resolved to understand more about English football if the back pages of the papers were to mean anything. Doreen Davies's words about understanding the British way of life were ringing in my ears.

Whilst working in Nottingham at Trent, I sought to soak up the atmosphere of the city by turning up at Forest matches, and I was also minded to watch Notts County play on the other side of the river. Although bearing the title of the oldest professional club in the world, the Magpies were then but a shadow of their 'Super Reds' rival carrying off all the trophies. Their ground at Meadow Lane was in a rather decrepit state, offering an opportunity, if you knew where to stand, to hear the manager's half-time talk to his players through the holes in the roof. Jimmy Sirrel's straight-talking, old-school words to his team were not great at most games, although that season did see some glimmers of hope.

My personal passion for British football came quickly. Having moved to London, I alighted on my local club Queens Park Rangers at the time Tommy Docherty was manager. *Shoot* magazine covered the occasion I even trained with them in 1979, with Gordon Hill, Tony Currie, David McCreery and Bob Hazell on-hand to offer expert advice, and the running and exercise routines supervised by Rangers assistant manager Ken Shellito. Picturing me sporting a blue Seventies tracksuit, the magazine declared that I 'could emerge as the superstar of the Radio 1 squad.'

I then dared to shift allegiance to Crystal Palace. Some fans never forgive a change in loyalties, even to a team in a division below rather than chasing success, but my genuine alibi was simply moving home to south-east London. I was also impressed by the welcome I received when helping with some charity proceedings at half-time at an Eagles match, with the atmosphere notably upbeat and family-friendly with a refreshingly high proportion of women in the crowd. I also confess to a preference for games played on grass pitches to the early artificial surfaces being adopted by several clubs at that time, with QPR leading the way with their Omniturf pitch laid in 1981.

At that stage, Steve Coppell was beginning his first spell as Palace manager, picking up from the rollercoaster ride of Allison, Venables and Kember, and it quickly became my team for life. I am president of the Crystal Palace Vice-President's Club; and acted as ambassador for the CPFC 2010 consortium when the club was being purchased from administrators. Our family became close, too, with the family of Ron Noades who, as chairman, was to lead the club through their brightest period.

My loyalty was repaid on my 40th birthday in 1990. Having driven home on a pleasant July night after hosting the drivetime show on Capital, I pulled the car into the driveway and noticed the roof of a marquee in our garden. It was not a surprise; ever the organiser, Guðrún had mentioned she might invite a few friends around.

On stepping foot in the front room, however, huge cheers and a bawdy rendition of 'Happy Birthday' rang out. Amongst other familiar faces, the entire Palace first team squad had descended to join my celebrations, notably Ian Wright, Mark Bright, John Salako, Andy Gray and Geoff Thomas, and their manager, the man who'd cleverly signed Ian from non-league football, Steve Coppell. Calling on her persuasive techniques, Guðrún had organised the touching affair secretly, knowing I would have been altogether more nervous about convening the occasion. They were all in high spirits, despite Palace's defeat in the FA Cup Final just weeks before. The birthday card signed by the lads was the biggest I had ever seen, bearing a menacing picture of a vulture, accompanied by suitably rude words bemoaning my age.

Upstairs, noises came from my daughter's bedroom. Pushing open the door, I caught sight of Mark Bright and Ian Wright sitting on her single bed; the partnership whose skills had made all the back pages with their goalscoring efforts for Crystal Palace in those late Eighties days. My daughter, it seemed, possessed the only working cassette player in the house, and the guys wanted to wallow in the radio commentary on their own matches from Capital's irrepressible Jonathan Pearce. In the days before 'Listen again', few players ever heard the shrieking excitement of radio commentary on their own goals.

The night's mood was to change rapidly. My birthday in July 1990 was also the date of the infamous England vs West Germany World Cup semi-final, played in Turin. The television in my house was turned up, and the players and other guests gathered around to witness a match which ended in penalties – and tears for England. Partying petered out.

Chris Tarrant had been in fine sprits, but his face fell flat. 'Are you still here?' he asked me in deadpan faux annoyance.

13

RADIO 1 IS WONDERFUL

As a topless Mick Jagger played with the Stones at the 1976 Knebworth festival in the hottest summer in living memory, I prepared to jump to the BBC.

Broadcasting House in London looms like a ship steaming down Portland Place. Walking through the original heavy revolving door, you heard the echoes of an Art Deco era as you passed under the eyes of the uniformed commissionaires and into a world of endless corridors and secret passages. In all the years I worked for the BBC, I could never walk into the foyer of that magisterial building without feeling the legacy of the dinner-jacketed announcers who had gone before.

BBC Radio 1 owned daytime pop radio in the UK in the Seventies. Thanks to a change in government, commercial radio's expansion was to be curtailed, serving only half the country. The BBC was largely alone, with Radio 1 audiences said to be over 20 million, delivered then on medium wave on a crackly 247 metres wavelength. Its music and familiar voices were heard in every home, car, shop and building site, laced with lush American jingles such as 'The Happy Sound of… Radio 1'.

The station's two studios were housed in what was the first floor of the old extension to Broadcasting House, alongside BBC Radio 2 and near the BBC Control Room. They were still referred to as 'cons', an abbreviation for 'continuities' as, when the station was hurriedly established, the studios used for the continuity announcements between programmes on the old Home Service,

Light and Third Programme were hastily converted into the 'self-op' studios demanded by the new breed of DJs. The impromptu arrangement lasted for almost twenty years.

As was the peculiar BBC tradition, faders on the studio mixing desk were pulled towards the operator, rather than pushed away, when a source of sound was required. Rumour has it the Corporation had favoured the topsy-turvy approach as it diminished the risk of the cufflinks of a formally-dressed announcer catching on a fader and airing something by accident. To me, it felt rather like driving a car on the wrong side of the road.

Predictably cueing up 'New Kid in Town' by the Eagles on the turntable on 25th September 1976, I nervously began my debut show on national UK radio, a Saturday morning affair billed in the *Radio Times* as 'Radio 1's new music man with two hours of the best sounds around.'

Welcome and generous encouragement came from the technical operators. Mike Hawkes was my producer in a programme which was to be billed, in time, as 'from punk to funk'. He selected the music and structured the ebb and flow of the show, although, as was the case with most presenters who were sufficiently interested in what they were playing, he allowed me to indulge in playing tracks I was particularly keen on; a freedom afforded nowadays to few daytime radio presenters.

The week prior, I had been a guest on Rosko's valedictory *Roundtable*. This hectic appearance was to be either the best or worst way of meeting my new colleagues, with almost the entire Radio 1 line-up taking turns to join us around the actual round table and vie for attention. An instruction to attend may have been issued by the boss, given John Peel, Paul Gambaccini, Alan Freeman, Tony Blackburn, Noel Edmonds, DLT, Ed Stewart and Savile all dutifully ventured into the studio to say hello to me and – more importantly – goodbye to Rosko.

Amidst the melee, I felt more relaxed than I had feared on opening my mouth for the first time on this huge radio station. Listening back now to recordings of that programme, I hear my enthusiasm for the latest release from the Scottish band Pilot, 'Penny In My Pocket', and my fears that they might have an 'image crisis'. In time, that song failed to chart. I also said I was not too impressed with re-issuing Motown hits, much preferring the new Supremes direction. Simon Bates disagreed, just prior to vacating his place round the table and stealing Rosko's cigarettes. Tony Blackburn enthused about the new song from Demis Roussos, 'When Forever Has Gone'. 'It'll be a big hit. A smash hit,' he said, and it was to prove another high-charting single for the Greek artist. I said I enjoyed the new David Essex single 'Coming Home', and suggested that of the male solo personalities in recent years, he rose above the rest, 'with standout and charisma.'

As *Roundtable* came to its end that day, there was little time to offer a full critical appraisal of the new release from the early-teens band Our Kid, the *New Faces* winners from Liverpool who had enjoyed success with 'You Just Might See Me Cry'. Noel suggested the shrill adolescent vocals actually belonged to Radio 1's new Kid. Lovely Alan Freeman was on good form on the show, seizing the opportunity to comment on the dark blue patch on the crutch of John Peel's jeans. It was a fitting, random introduction to my years at Radio 1.

The popular teen magazine *Jackie* enthusiastically covered my arrival with an article led by a puzzling photo of me sitting cross-legged on the floor beside shelves of LPs, mouth open wide in amazement and hands cupped needlessly round the headphones on my head. In the interview, I suggested that I did not object to still being 'Kid' despite being in my twenties, but added presumptuously that, like Bowie, people might just start to use my second name. I also seemed obsessed with response to a TV ad I had appeared in for a K-Tel album, the hugely popular Seventies compilations, commenting: 'The power of TV is staggering. People didn't associate me with *Rock On 45*, but they remember a 30-second commercial.'

On moving to London, we rented a flat in Hyde Park Square, acquiring fellow North American Paul Gambaccini as a neighbour. Always great company, and a consummate networker, he threw memorable parties including the one where caviar was served, picked from the sackful brought back from Russia by his friend. Being Paul, it had to be savoured in the proper fashion on Mother of Pearl spoons.

Our little tartan-collared white Westie grew to love his walks in Hyde Park, where we regularly bumped into *Man About the House* actor Yootha 'Mildred Roper' Joyce walking her Pekinese. Arrow was our dog's name, borrowed from the song 'Me and My Arrow' from Harry Nilsson's 1971 album *The Point!* Given to us as a wedding present, Arrow came as an unwelcome surprise initially to Guðrún, who had been brought up in Reykjavík where dogs were not allowed until 1984.

At the time Radio 1 was still joined at the hip with Radio 2, so 'Diddy' David Hamilton was squatting across both stations each weekday afternoon, amassing formidable audiences. It was impossible to scan up and down long wave, medium wave or FM without being greeted by his warm tones.

Johnnie Walker had just left the station on a matter of principle, displeased at being told his contract would be renewed only if he undertook to play fewer album tracks, and thus, by implication, more singles including the likes of the Bay City Rollers, whom he had referred to as 'musical garbage'.

By contrast, Punk was beginning to make its mark both as a musical genre and a cultural phenomenon, and I loved its energy and spirit. How invigorating to witness the likes of the Cure or Siouxsie and the Banshees live and, particularly, the Clash, whose first gig was supporting the Sex Pistols in Sheffield with the excellent Joe Strummer as frontman. Ian Dury encouraged me to invite them on to the programme, assuring me that despite their defiant image they were the sort of principled guys who never let you down, always showing up for their friends when needed. On the first occasion we met, they all duly showed up and we crammed into a small room to record a hugely-engaging and candid conversation that started a friendship which has endured. I found them the real deal, with so much more to offer than relentless punk viciousness.

John Peel was reportedly less impressed by them, commenting: 'The Clash did half a session and then wandered off – unbearably pretentious.'[11] Whilst the two sides of the story of that unfinished session will now never be heard, it's unlikely John was enamoured with Joe Strummer's comments, reported in the *NME*, that: 'listening to John Peel was like a dog being sick in your face.'[12]

Derek Chinnery controlled Radio 1 from 1979 to 1985; a man with a real presence, well-regarded by the BBC. Honest, yet polite, reserved and strait-laced, you were sure to check there were no holes in your jeans before calling in to his office for a meeting. Hearing the music John Peel played and then looking at Derek, John's ultimate boss, it was difficult to countenance quite how the two co-existed. They did, thanks to Derek's trust in Peel's producer John Walters, who famously said: 'Working with Peel is like taking a dog for a walk; you just have to make sure he doesn't cock his leg at any musical lamp-post for too long.'[13]

As with many young newcomers to any radio station, I was charged initially with filling the shoes of holidaying presenters in my early days at Radio 1. The short 'depping' stints afford new recruits a useful opportunity to become familiar gently with the station, with the limited exposure risking little long-term

11 www.bbc.co.uk/radio1/mostpunk/peel_sessions.shtml.
12 *NME*, March 1991.
13 John Walters obituary by Chris Lycett, *The Guardian*, 1st August 2000.

audience damage if things fall apart.

To be invited to play the part of Noel Edmonds on the Radio 1 Breakfast Show, however, seemed rather like asking me to jump from 5-a-side to playing midfielder for England. The programme had been under Noel's captaincy since Tony Blackburn moved to the mid-morning slot in 1973. Its scale and reputation were daunting, but in 1977 I was asked to do my best and wake up Britain for three weeks.

Marc Bolan's death added to the pressure. The flamboyant front man for T. Rex lost his life aged just 29 in the early hours of 16th of September 1977, during my first week deputising, when the Mini in which he was travelling crashed into a tree on Barnes Common. 'Too beautiful to live, too young to die,' as he used to say; and to this day, a huge patch of fresh flowers always marks the spot. All broadcasters are familiar with the challenge of tailoring the mood of a programme when your audience is just coming to terms with the death of a figure who has meant much to them. Marc and I first met early in his career when he appeared on my TV show *45*; indeed, his own show *Marc* replaced it, also produced by Muriel Young in Manchester. He had been a friend of John Peel, although that relationship became prickly as Marc's profile soared. I found him self-assured, although that is neither an undesirable nor unusual trait in a performer of his nature.

Dave Lee Travis (DLT) eventually succeeded Noel as the Breakfast Show's permanent host, becoming known as the Hairy Cornflake, and the resultant programme shuffle meant I was asked to assume his old show in spring 1978. He had referred to it as the 'teatime show', whilst the *Radio Times* dubbed it *It's DLT OK!*. In its early days, the programme ended at 7.30, with an uncomfortable juxtaposition as Radio 1 joined with a then mellow Radio 2, and hits from the likes of Suzi Quatro collided with melodies from the Scottish Radio Orchestra.

The Friday edition of my new programme included Rosko's

former feature, *Roundtable*. Over the years its guest list of music icons was impressive, both from the UK and the US, and Annie Nightingale was known to linger to capture photos of the weekly encounters.

On one occasion I shared a lift to the studio with Chrissie Hynde, whom I simply adored, quaking at the knees as we scaled the storeys when this artist, whose talent, voice and look I admired so much, put her arm into mine.

Al Stewart, from Los Angeles, produced some impressive folk-rock material in the Seventies, with albums such as *Time Passages* and *Year of the Cat*. When he appeared on *Roundtable* he mentioned the winery he owned in California, and even brought in a couple of bottles of Chateau Margaux 1966, worth many hundreds of pounds. The fine claret tasted and smelt like Christmas, despite our glugging it in the studio from some of the old BBC cardboard cups.

The programme's Hall of Fame included other such names as Ian Dury, Kate Bush, Lionel Richie, Nick Lowe, Steve Harley, Debbie Harry, Elvis Costello, Leo Sayer, B.B. King, Dusty Springfield, Lene Lovich, Francis Rossi, Justin Hayward and Herb Alpert.

Given the format revolved around an honest critique of the passionate labours of other artists, there was always the risk of causing offence. The US group Kid Creole and the Coconuts had enjoyed a string of deserving Top Ten hits in the Eighties, but I felt the new release we reviewed on *Roundtable* did not quite hit the mark. I said as much on-air, amplifying comments I had penned for my *Melody Maker* column. The following week, midway through a song, the studio door barged open and in walked their manager Randy Hoffman, his assistant and three mean-looking guys, suggesting they 'wanted a word' about what I had said. Bearing the expression of a frightened man I looked around in panic, until eventually their faces broke into laughter. It had been a highly effective wind-up – but I do not recall troubling to review any further singles from the group.

In various hands, *Roundtable* had featured in the Radio 1 programme schedule from 1970, before being laid to rest in the mid-Eighties. I enjoyed my spell hugely, as the format afforded the time for real insight into the guests' personalities and knowledge as they spoke at length of things other than their own music.

Best friends can be honest enough to offer the best advice in the most constructive way. Paul Burnett volunteered some valuable criticism, having appeared as a guest on the programme, when he observed how often my gaze shifted away from the interviewee whilst I chatted, preferring to look with seeming urgency at the cartridge tape players, my notes, the clock, or the turntables instead. He correctly identified that the trait was more through habit than necessity, and illustrated how it feels as a guest to have a question posed only for the interviewer to look away promptly in seeming disinterest. His point was thoroughly valid, as illustrated vividly many years later when my Harley Street consultant shuffled his papers on his desk rather than look me in the eye.

Newsbeat was Radio 1's extended news programme, airing daily at lunchtime and at 5.30. Whilst it had merit, its scheduling was slightly uncomfortable, interrupting the flow of music in my programme just as the momentum was beginning to build. It did, however, allow a welcome break and coincided with a visit from the regular BBC 'tea lady', a ritual which was exactly as you would imagine. She arrived on schedule, pushing a tea trolley bearing cups and saucers and a large Corporation-coloured china teapot.

Years later, as I prepared to host an edition of *Top of the Pops*, one of the artists came up to me. 'You don't remember me, do you?' I confessed not, until she helpfully reminded me of her Lincolnshire roots. Only then did it dawn on me that my BBC tea lady was now about to perform her Number Four chart hit. Corinne Drewery from Swing Out Sister patiently explained how her trademark dark bob hairstyle had now replaced the long locks which would have been more familiar to me from her trolley-pushing days.

Another TV opportunity, featuring contestants from different ITV regions, surfaced in 1976. Initiated by Ian Bolt from Yorkshire TV, *Pop Quest* saw me sitting on a futuristic set marshalling a *University Challenge*-type format in which long-haired teens chewed gum and answered questions on music and charts to win guitars, sound equipment or just a record token.

The wonderfully funny Sally James co-hosted the quiz show with me, just before and during her days alongside Chris Tarrant on the children's Saturday morning show *TISWAS*. I hopped on an early train north to record *Pop Quest* for its Friday transmission, and enjoyed the customary marmalade breakfast en-route. Despite their typical tardiness, to this Canadian there was always something romantic about those journeys.

Radio 1 carried particular responsibilities as a public service broadcaster and tried to meet them in a way which suited the audience, so a cluster of major features were installed at the tail-end of my show, referred to stuffily in the BBC's annual report as 'spoken word items… of interest to young people.'[14] Although I had built my career in music radio, I cultivated many other interests and it was refreshing to have good excuse to attack a range of topics on-air.

In-depth artist interviews were amongst the features. Billy Joel was one candidate in 1983, who requested we share a bottle of port to accompany the discussion about his new album *An Innocent Man*. I drank very slowly.

The same year, David Bowie, then aged 36 and looking fit and tanned from the Australian sunshine, called in for an oft-quoted, generally jovial appearance when promoting *Let's Dance*. Outspoken about his former record company RCA, he opined

---

14 *BBC Annual Report and Handbook, 1985.*

that 'the belief had gone in each other,' and that there was 'no love lost between us.' The compilation albums they had assembled were dubbed 'horrendous' and 'most offensive', sounding 'like they were done over half an hour in a board meeting.' When probed about future collaborations, he said he had 'never really wanted to record with other people', although he conceded that working with the pioneering German electronic band Kraftwerk would be fun.

Bowie confessed there were some items of memorabilia from his career he felt he could not bear to throw out, including his Stylophone – the miniature stylus-operated keyboard instrument he had played on 'Space Oddity', and he had certainly treasured 'every item of clothing I've ever worn', including the *Ziggy Stardust* costumes from Japanese designer Kansai Yamamoto.

My evening programme included *Kid's Mailbag*, based on a US show called *You Asked for It* which had begun in the late 1950s. Our interpretation generated a huge volume of letters, in which curious listeners asked us to solve questions or challenges. In those pre-Wikipedia days, we were sent queries like 'How do they get lead into pencils?', and sought to answer them with such devices as, in that case, a response from an earnest expert at a pencil museum. In the days before eBay, too, many questions were received about the value of records or treasured autographed photographs. Bonhams, the auctioneers, contributed solutions regularly, and it was fascinating to witness the value of celebrity memorabilia rise and fall in line with the ebb and flow of their fame. Those changing values were perhaps a lesson for all of us in the public eye. My producer Dave Tate and I sifted through the piles of puzzled mail for the most compelling topics, and he efficiently sourced the answers ready for the show.

Alison Rice joined me for the *Girl Talk* segment, which evolved into talk about world travel, a topic for which she later gained recognition on TV-am, and *Staying Alive* featured reassurance to worried young listeners from Dr Alan Maryon-Davis in response to questions about their bodies. As one programme trailer boasted: 'Tonight at 7, Colin Hall-Dexter from the British Dental Health Foundation. So, if you fancy some talk about teeth, join us.'

Your Chance to Meet a Sportsman offered an opportunity to interview major names from the sporting world such as Nigel Mansell, Mike Brearley and Mario Andretti. It was a coup to feature Joe Bugner the night before his famous heavyweight clash with Richard Dunn in October 1976 at Wembley for the Commonwealth and European belts. Whilst we visited most interviewees on their home turf, Bugner willingly came into the studio to record the piece. Seeming on excellent form, chatting readily about anything that crossed his mind, the interview gave a surprisingly honest insight into the man. His language was natural and colourful, but there was little which could not be made ready for broadcast with a few judicious edits. At the end of the interview we discovered the reason for the candid conversation, when he declared 'Right, I'm ready to get started now.' The next evening Bugner knocked out Dunn in the first round.

Johnny Beerling was my senior producer, later to take over the overall management of Radio 1 from Derek Chinnery. His controllership in 1985 was the right appointment at the right time – a doer and a fixer with the knack of getting things organised in an organisation which might otherwise be less agile. Johnny is credited as having steered Radio 1 through a hugely-successful spell.

We got on well and shared a love of motorsports, both looking forward to the Radio 1 Fun Days at race meetings, with the first being staged at Brands Hatch where presenters careered around the track in souped-up Ford Mexicos. Such daring was a feature of Radio 1's image of the time, as demonstrated in 1978 when daredevil stunt performer Eddie Kidd planned to ride his motorcycle over ten Radio 1 presenters laid end-to-end on the ground at Brands Hatch. I was positioned closest to the safety of the ramp, although there was still genuine risk from the 80mph world record attempt. Aside from my own safety, it crossed my mind that Johnny Beerling would be highly upset were I injured given that the Radio 1 calendar for 1979 had already been printed – and I was the December pinup. As at many stations in the uncertain world of radio, a star position in the annual merchandising plan was a decent indication of how secure your job was.

On one occasion at Brands Hatch, Paul Gambaccini 'raced' Annie Nightingale on push scooters. He remembers that whilst sitting in the Grovewood hospitality suite awaiting our turn, and watching our colleagues do all manner of puzzling things that did not interest us hugely, I observed: 'This is the only reality. Everything else is a dream.'

At another of the race days, Johnny observed the gifts of a good-looking blond young man called Mike Smith, who was compering the day; talent-spotting which led to Mike's appointment at Radio 1, where he would later host the Breakfast Show.

Treasured grainy Polaroid shots of huge crowds of Radio 1 listeners cheering on hot, sunny days at the coast tell the colourful story of another of Johnny's clever initiatives – the famous Radio 1 Roadshow, which began with Alan Freeman from Newquay in 1973. The red, white and blue cavalcade descended on resorts and other carefully chosen locations dotted around the UK, and we looned about in front of those who had made their way to see us. On the warmest days, attendance numbered many thousands, with queues battling to access the resort and children hoisted onto parents' shoulders to watch our antics and shout until they were hoarse. Smiley Miley sold off his popular mugs and T-shirts so the kids could leave the packed fields clutching a souvenir. Those attending in their youth likely remember those occasions to this day.

The enjoyment was mutual, and Radio 1 presenters were always keen for the coveted summer rota to appear. In the late Seventies, I took to the Roadshow stage in Portsmouth, Tenby, Bournemouth, Weymouth, Morecambe, Exmouth and Colwyn Bay.

In its early days, music acts were not an integral part of the offering, and it is puzzling that so many listeners made so much effort just to come to see a guy in a field playing records.

As the concept matured and its infrastructure grew, major acts were scheduled to appear with us, with Wham! and the Belle Stars sharing the stage with me at South Park during the Macclesfield carnival, where the clamour for autographs from banner-waving fans turned into madness. I dared to venture into the crowd to risk some live on-air dedications, which were just audible over the noise. 'What do you like best about the carnival?' I asked one festival-goer. 'Not much,' she replied. The event was challenging from the outset, and was only made possible by the generosity of neighbours as our engineers dangled a power cable across the lake and plugged it into the power supply of a nearby house.

In Cleethorpes, more than seven thousand people came to see us in 1983 when Spandau Ballet arrived by helicopter to join us at the boating lake paddock. Some dedicated fans arrived just after dawn to be sure of a place at the front, from where they were even treated to the sight of band members on board the miniature railway.

The Radio 1 team spent time together on these occasions and, albeit for a short spell, there was more of the familiar Radio Luxembourg prankster spirit. On that occasion on the north-east coast, I was handcuffed to a barrier until I agreed to forsake my trousers for a pair of shorts.

One Roadshow took me to Whitley Bay and, as always, we lingered after the show near our promotional caravan to chat to visitors and sign autographs. Three very polite young men approached me and handed over a tape, explaining they were in a band and pleading with me to listen to their work. Slotting the cassette into the player on the long drive back south, it impressed immediately and I promptly tried to arrange for them to record a Radio 1 session. It was after airing some of that material one night on the show that a call came from Steve Winwood's brother Muff, then head of A&R at Columbia Records. The rest is history – for the stylish Prefab Sprout. In my December 1983 *Daily Mirror* column predicting the stars of 1984, I enthused: 'The delicate acoustic style, married to weird, wonderful words and the voices of Paddy McAloon and Wendy Smith will make listening to their debut album, *Swoon*, due out in March, a heady experience.'

Another landmark roadshow took us to Ulster at a sensitive time in history. Plans were carefully scrutinised, although the head of BBC Northern Ireland was confident that the event would proceed safely. With sensible security measures in place, I was installed in the impressive Culloden Hotel just outside the city, in the suite usually commanded by Home Secretary William Whitelaw. Ironically, no-one seemed to have noticed the lock on the door barely functioned. Against the backdrop of the Troubles, I was struck by the warmth of the welcome at what was then the New University of Ulster, and how friendly people were. Johnny Beerling, who produced the show personally, recalled in his 2008 book the enthusiastic crowd of three thousand listeners at the roadshow, and the staging of a Captain Sensible lookalike contest on-stage, with the aid of oversized spectacles as props.[15]

Just as *Blue Peter* presenters were instructed by the formidable Biddy Baxter to wear their badges on screen, it was insisted upon that we wear the vibrant red, white and blue Radio 1 jackets bearing our names when out on show together. The uniform did help us look like a family, which is possibly what the listeners of

15 *Radio 1: The Inside Scene*, Johnny Beerling.

the time wanted and expected.

My jacket was eventually donated to a girl whose listening loyalty extended to her waiting for us to finish our programmes at Broadcasting House, just so she could catch a glimpse of her heroes on the way out. As I walked past her one day, I took off my well-worn coat and draped it around her shoulders. Wherever she is, I hope she remembers that day even now – although I suspect she ditched the jacket long ago.

The team also united for the Radio 1 Week Out, where a town or city was adopted as a station base for the whole week. It was sometimes suggested with a smile that the spread of locations we identified appeared to bear some resemblance to the early map of commercial radio stations. A host of events were devised each day, with many hours of programming from shop windows, restaurants and canteens, rounded off with charity fundraising and gigs, attracting ready support from top-rank acts. Returning to their home turf, the Undertones performed a set in Northern Ireland, and ABC joined us in Sheffield. I had championed the Pretenders in their earliest days, so it was great to see them turn up in Cardiff to perform a set at Glan Ely High School. What a tremendous opportunity for the pupils – and teachers – to have a band of that calibre in their school hall. Elvis never dropped in to my school assembly.

At the time of that performance in the late Seventies, the Pretenders' track 'Kid' was a hit, and one of the band suggested it was inspired by my nickname. Chrissie Hynde smiled in agreement, and told me she had written it after reading an article about me in *Here's Health* magazine. I suspect they were having a joke at my expense, but I choose to believe, nevertheless.

The Week Out initiative routinely kicked off on the Sunday night with a football match between Radio 1 and a celebrity team from the host town. For us, it was a laugh and a way of getting to know the community, but the opposing teams took things more seriously, often intent on annihilation by recruiting determined ex-pros to bolster their chances. When a ball was hurled into your stomach, you knew about it. I got through the matches by dreaming that I was playing for Crystal Palace, which made the considerable aches afterwards worthwhile. As Paul Gambaccini reminded me, 'We were both inept, of course, having grown up in countries where football was referred to as "soccer", and was usually limited to elite schools.'

John Inverdale, now recognised as an accomplished sports broadcaster, was head of student union activities at the University of Southampton in the Seventies, and he choreographed our visit there in 1978. My programme was broadcast live, but that evening sticks in my mind not for the fine welcome we received but for the Tuesday evening ritual of the chart recap. As I reached for the piece of paper bearing the Top Twenty listing, it was handed to me by naughty Noel, who had set fire to the bottom of it with a cigarette lighter. The burning script is the oldest slapstick joke in the radio book, but never fails. It prompted me to deliver the chart rundown at an ever-growing pace before the whole page turned to ash.

At many radio stations, the team of presenters are regularly summoned to lively gatherings at base to be briefed on the latest news and plans, rounded off with a little rabble-rousing. It was never like that at Radio 1. Although we had pride in what we achieved, we each worked at different times of the day, scattered across the BBC's rambling premises, and were routinely whisked off site to deal with all the other related work of assorted voiceovers, TV and public appearances. Unlike the confinement of Radio Luxembourg, we lived our own lives with our own families and social circles, and we had grown up, so had little time for the sort of jokes we had played at Radio Luxembourg.

Johnnie Walker and DLT were both good to me on my arrival at Radio 1, helping me settle in London, and it was pleasing to meet up with Noel again, who had left Luxembourg the year after I arrived. Although always busy with his various entrepreneurial ventures, he and I and our wives used to enjoy a meal out together on many occasions. Each of us had friends in the Radio 1 team to whom we grew close, alongside those with whom we simply had perfectly decent professional relations. As might be expected, however, there were also competitive elements and a degree of friction between individual team members, so the flavour of some pranks could be rather different from those at 208.

John Peel and Simon Bates were not cut from the same cloth, and I remember the occasion when John returned from the McDonalds near Oxford Circus with a milkshake, only to blow the contents of it into Simon's locker through a straw poking through the keyhole. On another occasion I was drawn reluctantly into a plot with him to bend back the windscreen wipers on Simon's car. Having traipsed downstairs to the basement car park, I pointed out the CCTV cameras – and the plan was wisely aborted.

Down the corridor from the individual offices lay the open-plan area where the hard-working secretaries were perched at their desks, opening mail, dealing with calls, and typing what needed to be typed on their clattering manual typewriters. Although the administration staff were friendly and clearly relished the role they played at the entertainment end of the BBC's operation, I always felt intimidated by them, albeit with no justification. Much to the amusement of a puzzled Paul Burnett, I passed their desks only when necessary, gliding by with head down, hoping not to be noticed. Although more self-assured on the surface than I had been at Luxembourg, I was still shy. Many broadcasters are similarly reserved, which comes as a surprise to many who witness us performing to crowds of thousands and audiences of millions. The paradox extends to entertainers too: who would recognise the quiet and modest Jimi Hendrix I interviewed from the image of his guitar-burning on-stage persona? I try not to allow myself to get nervous, but like many of us I am less daunted by walking out on stage to thousands of anonymous faces than talking to a small audience of faces I recognise.

Radio 1 adopted the Royal Variety Club as its nominated charity, supporting its efforts extensively and helping it fund the Sunshine Coaches to provide much-needed transport for children with disabilities. In turn, their local branches often supported our activities across the country. It was at a Variety Club fundraiser that I first met Eric Morecambe, one of the revered British comedy icons with whom I quickly had to familiarise myself when moving to the UK. The early appearances of Morecambe and Wise on the *Ed Sullivan Show* in the US from 1963 to 1968 had been a puzzle to viewers that side of the World, with the suited duo appearing so different from their home-grown performers.

On watching Eric at ease at the Variety Club function in London, it was clear he was one of those comedians who was just effortlessly funny. As we were being positioned carefully for a group photograph, I was asked to kneel at the front of the shot, with Eric standing behind. Instinctively seizing the comedy in the moment, he placed both his legs over my shoulders, as if riding a horse. Then, preening himself, he looked around, paused and said to me: 'All right, cock?' It is not funny – but it is when he does it. Anyone who knows Morecambe and Wise can picture his black spectacles, his expression, his delivery, and the impeccable timing of that simple remark and appreciate just how gifted he was.

The efforts of the Variety Club extended to sponsoring a sports luncheon in 1984 for Outward Bound, the charity whose mission is to inspire young people to defy their limitations. Prince Philip was then its patron, which led to my being asked to interview His Royal Highness. Despite all the usual preparatory Royal rigmarole, he was typically relaxed once on microphone. In a wry aside, he suggested that 'The fascinating thing about the British is that they can really only enjoy themselves thoroughly if they are giving some money for charity. In some way, it salves their conscience.' Listening back to the interview now, I hear myself trying valiantly to sound as English as I possibly could.

A puzzling request for an appearance came from the American actor Lauren Bacall, a huge star of classic Hollywood cinema who played alongside the likes of Marilyn Monroe. For reasons that are beyond me, her agent requested my services for the launch of Lauren's new cosmetics range at the Royal Festival Hall. As I stood at the lectern extolling the virtues of some moisturiser, I picked her face out in the crowd, sitting in an aisle seat, her legs crossed. She was looking at me. I returned the gaze, staring into the eyes which had stared at her husband – Humphrey Bogart.

Being in the public eye runs the risk of starring in inadvertent headlines. After a successful gig in Berkshire, I was perplexed to see the *Daily Star* reporting next day: 'Police to interview DJ about murder'. The article reported that there had been a knife incident at a gig I had happened to host the previous night, and suggested I might hold the key to a murderer's identity. I knew nothing of said crime, nor was I ever interrogated by the local constabulary. Just my being there that night seemed to be sufficient for a journalist to splice me into a tragic story.

○

Society might have benefited from Savile featuring in headlines earlier than he did. Every memory of him is now viewed through the lens of the appalling crimes he committed. Whilst his face appears in several much-used Radio 1 group photographs, he was not on the daily schedule and was rarely seen at the station, as many of my colleagues will testify. In my time, his voice was heard on his odd *Old Record Club* programmes on Sunday which were recorded off-site.

He did turn up at a Radio 1 Christmas party one year, held at the home of the then boss, Derek Chinnery. As I was chatting with Paul Burnett about Elvis's death, Savile interrupted to insist how close he had been to the King, and proceeded to regale us with his conspiracy theories about his premature end.

On that occasion, and others, I had little idea what he was talking about. I concluded the odd yodelling noise he made was just a device he used to fill the awkward silence. Self-obsessed, he had little to say about anything or anybody else. If out in public when not on duty, he wore wigs and strange clothes as a disguise to avoid being spoken to, but at the BBC, it was easy for him to keep himself to himself, because no-one wanted to talk to him. He was not one of us.

Standing outside Broadcasting House one day chatting to Derek Chinnery, we noticed two limousines pull up. Savile walked across and climbed into the rear car. 'Evening professors,' he said as he slid into the back seat, holding his cigar. The first car pulled off, followed by the second as he was driven away. Derek explained that when Savile had an important appointment, he had heard he took two vehicles as a precaution lest one broke down.

He was a bright guy who used that asset selfishly, engineering several quiet product endorsement deals. His own PR efficiency ensured his 'charity work' was always recognised, and many at the station were disdainful of his efforts in seeking so much attention for them. We now know more about the darkness of the distraction he was engineering around him. When stories about alleged misdemeanours – and I heard nothing more serious than that – were gossiped about, they were often attributed to people being jealous of his profile.

Despite his many *NME* Top DJ awards – every year from 1964 to 1972 – he was certainly never that.

Savile was odd, and, as we now know, a criminal of the worst kind, leaving an appalling trail of victims whose stories of suffering were listened to too late. His appalling behaviour has also tainted a generation's memories, and has diminished the achievements of all who happened to be at Radio 1 when his name was on the schedule.

○

Inch by inch, Radio 1 was cutting the apron strings from Radio 2 and growing into a full-time service. Radio 2 itself was also planning to expand into round-the-clock programming, then a rarity in UK radio. The plans were thwarted, however, in the winter of 1978 owing to industrial action by the Association of Broadcasting Staff. For a short spell, all BBC radio networks fused in a way usually reserved for the most dramatic of national emergencies. Yet again, I was on-air at the time, albeit with none of the drama of the Radio Trent strike debacle. It did mean that I was heard simultaneously on Radio 1, 2, 3 and 4, declaring 'This is the BBC Radio All Network Service – and I'm Kid Jensen.' My programme followed Radio 2's calm John Dunn and a puzzled news bulletin delivered by the fruity tones of Brian Perkins, who wryly observed my appearance on the Radio 3 transmitters. The issue of BBC pay parity with ITV workers was settled just in time for Christmas, with the press reporting that radio was 'back to normal' and television screens would be carrying the Corporation's key festive fixture – the first televising of *The Sound of Music*.

The business of radio can become a serious affair, but, as presenters, we felt largely insulated from any serious Corporation concerns being chewed over in oak-panelled rooms elsewhere at Broadcasting House. As the station's executive producer the buck stopped with Johnny Beerling, who probably shielded us from some of the Corporation's less sensible demands of its pop channel. He understood us and our work, and understandably seemed more at home being hands-on making radio than sitting in on meetings. Even as commercial radio took its tentative first steps, during my first spell at Radio 1 I got the impression that the prospect of competition did not generally seem to pre-occupy middle-management overmuch. Whilst there was a growing professionalism and focus, the station wisely seemed to me to devote its energies to itself, not the competition.

Further up the management tree, the BBC indicated more suspicion about the activities of the new commercial entrants. A handful of Radio 1 DJs were summoned on one occasion for a lunch with Aubrey Singer, then managing director of all BBC radio. We gathered at the excellent L'Etoile in Charlotte Street, curious of the agenda, only to find that Aubrey was seeking our views on Capital Radio. We discussed its excellent music, presenters and general culture, for which there was genuine respect, and the Help a London Child appeal which had been running since 1975. Aubrey seemed particularly fascinated by the impact of the huge fundraiser which seemed to be the talk of London every Easter. I can never be sure, but it would be good to think that our lunch with a pretender to the DG's crown was one of the catalysts for the BBC's Children in Need appeal.

The most welcome surprise about that get-together was that our views were valued. A key BBC apparatchik had troubled to ask us what we thought – an approach which contrasted starkly with that of other bosses I would encounter in my later career who would find it utterly impossible to countenance that any DJ could possibly have any intelligent contribution to make in any matter.

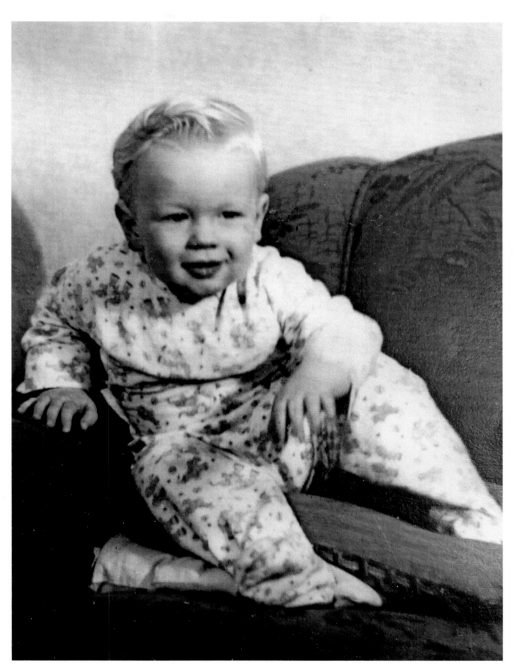

1. Christmas 1951

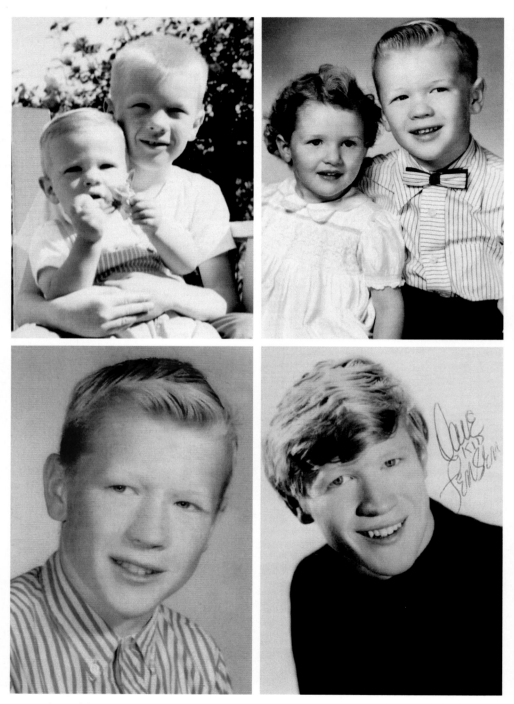

2. Four faces of the Kid...
Top left: With brother Lee. Top right: Wiith sister Linda
Bottom left: Aged 10. Bottom right: Early Radio Luxembourg promo card

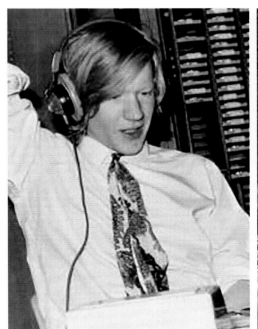
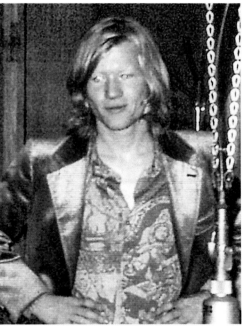

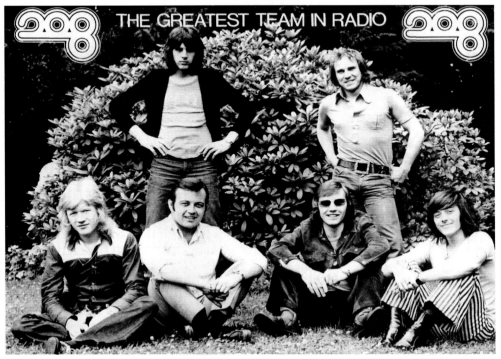

THE GREATEST TEAM IN RADIO

3. Young star of Radio Luxembourg 208, 'the greatest team in radio'.
Courtesy Honey Bee Benson

4. Luxy days: a star is born.

Bottom: Kid joins Noddy Holder and Don Powell of Slade in saluting Thin Lizzy at the London Rainbow, November 1972.

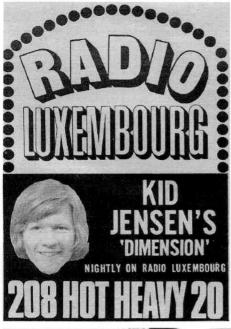

RADIO LUXEMBOURG

KID JENSEN'S 'DIMENSION'

NIGHTLY ON RADIO LUXEMBOURG

208 HOT HEAVY 20

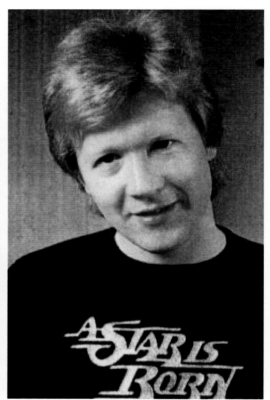

A STAR IS BORN

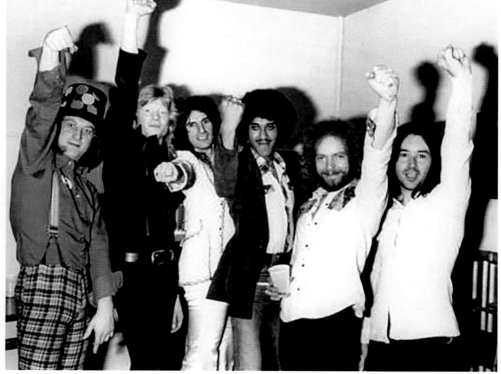

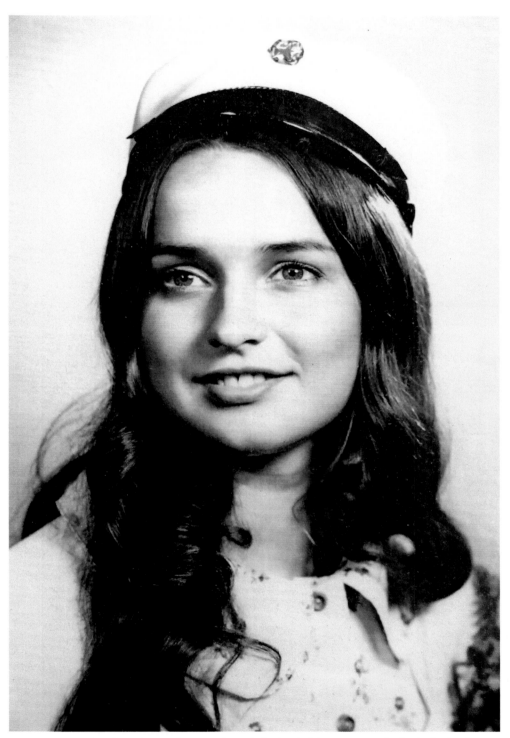

5. Guðrún's graduation from Verslunarskoli Islands (The Commercial School of Iceland), 1973

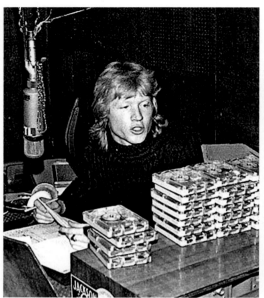

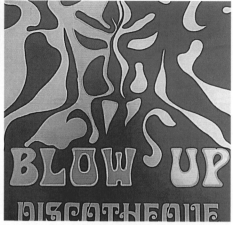

6. *Jensen's Dimensions.*
Bottom: At the Blow Up with Mark Wesley and Tony Prince
Courtesy Honey Bee Benson

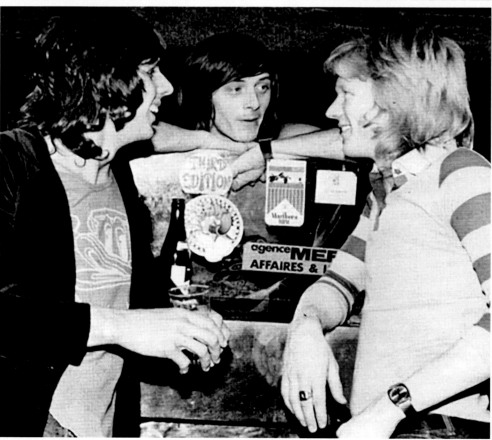

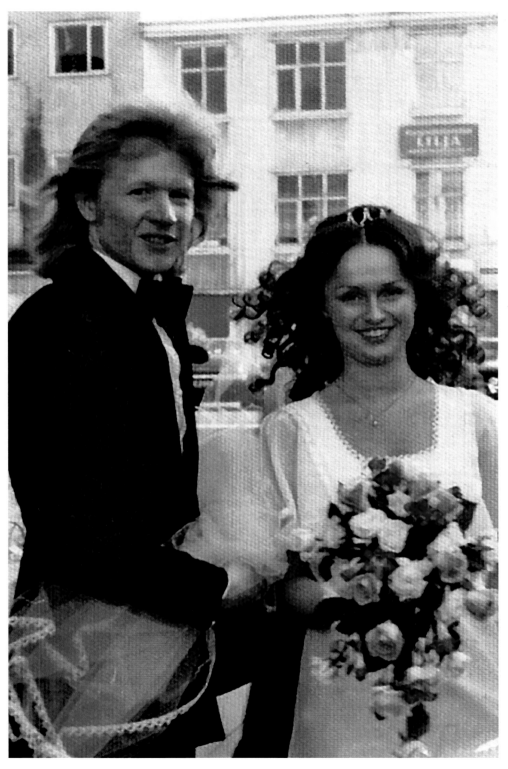

7. Reykjavík, June 1975

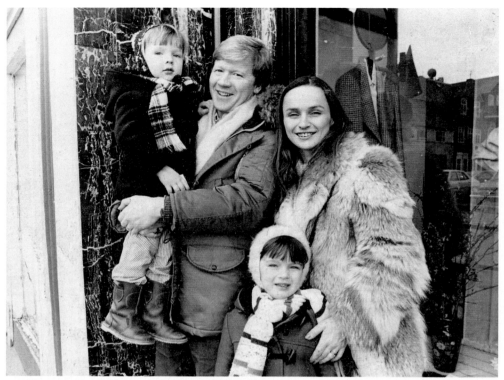

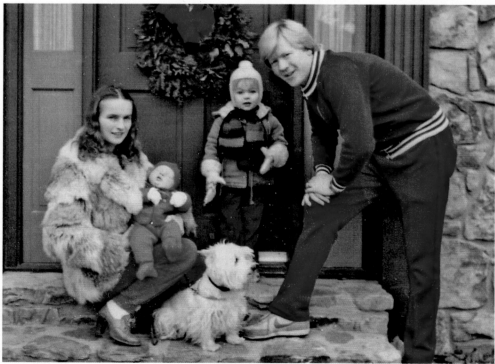

8. Top: With Anna Lisa and Alexander in Iceland
Bottom: A family Christmas in Atlanta, Georgia

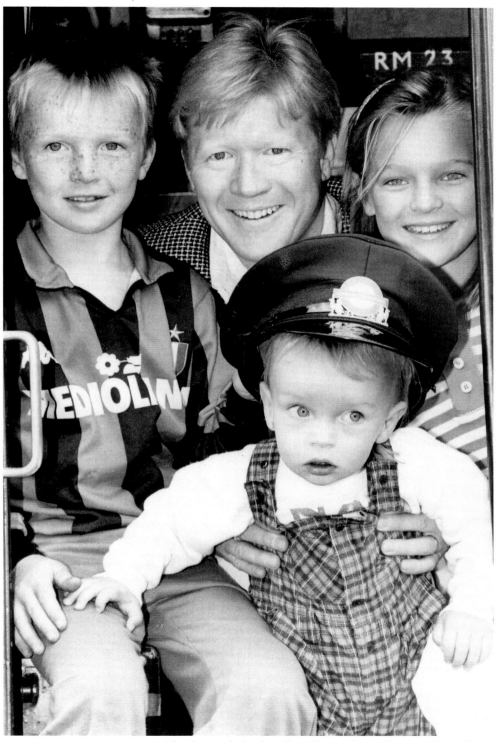

9. After driving the last bus along Clarence Street, Kingston-Upon-Thames before it was pedestrianised, with a little help from conductor Viktor Thor

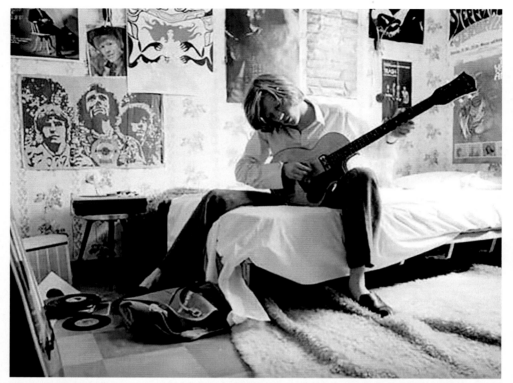

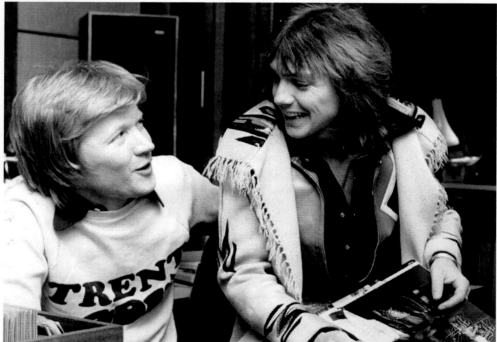

10. Top: The Rocker
Bottom: With David Cassidy at Radio Trent, 1976
Courtesy Honey Bee Benson

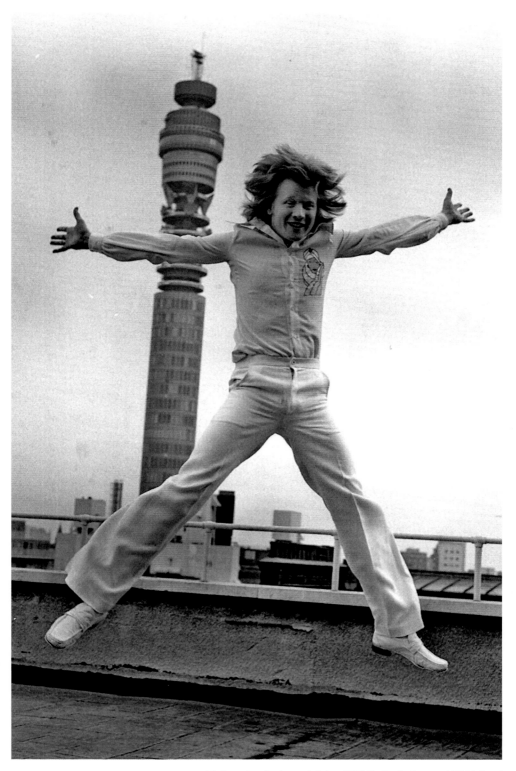

11. Jumping for joy at joining BBC Radio 1, August 1976 (Alamy)

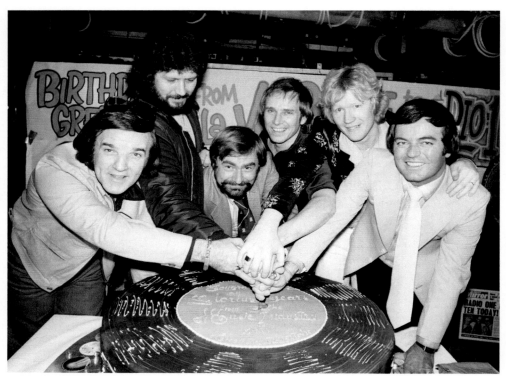

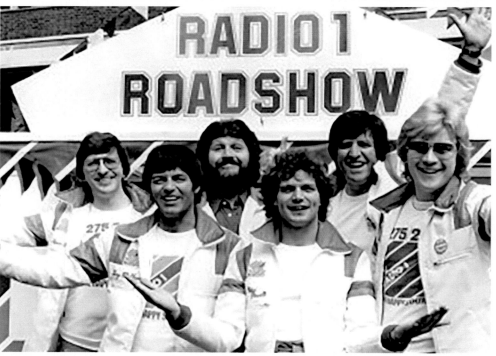

11. Top: (L-R) Alan Freeman, Dave Lee Travis. Paul Gambaccini, Adrian Juste,
Kid and Tony Blackburn celebrate ten years of Radio 1 (Alamy)
Bottom: Simon Bates, Tony Blackburn, DLT, Peter Powell, Ed Stewart and Kid take a trip to the seaside

12. Top: (left) "It's the Kid!" (right) Top of the Pops with Kate Bush (Alamy)
Bottom: Michael Jackson and George Harrison flank Kid and his producer, Mike Hawkes (BBC)

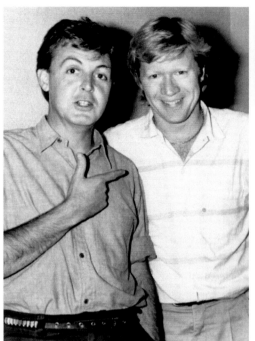

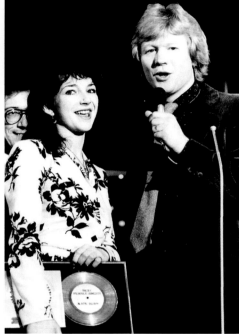

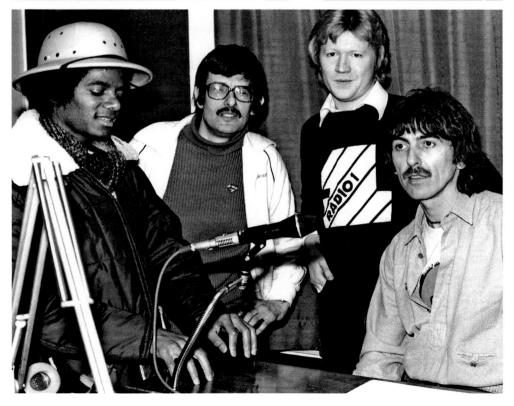

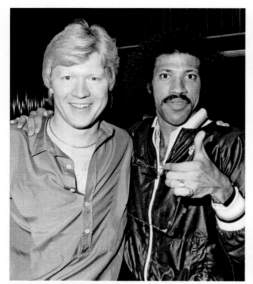 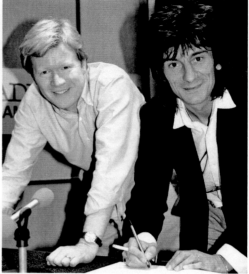

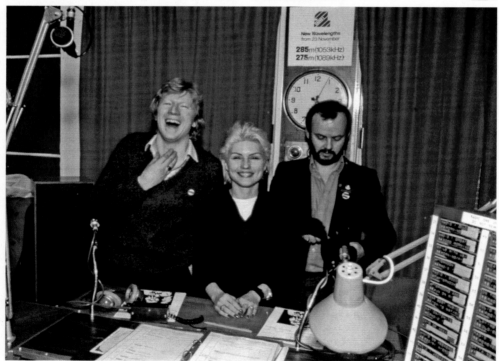

13. Top: (left) Hello! With Lionel Richie (right) Rollin' with Ronnie Wood
Bottom: Debbie Harry entertains the Rhythm Pals (BBC)

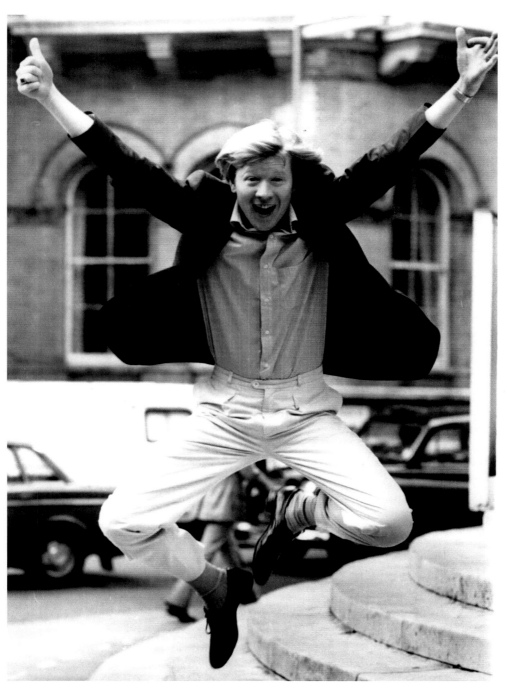

14. Jumping for joy at joining TBS for a new adventure in America, May 1980 (Alamy)

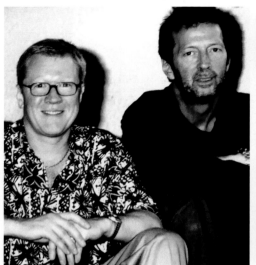
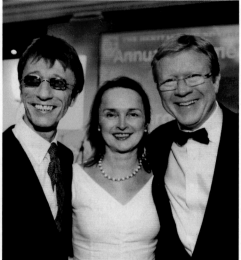
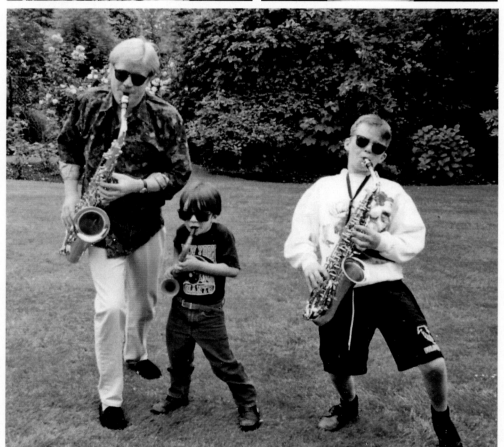

15. *Top: (left) Slowhand (right) With Robin Gibb*
Bottom: The Jensen Saxophone Trio warm up

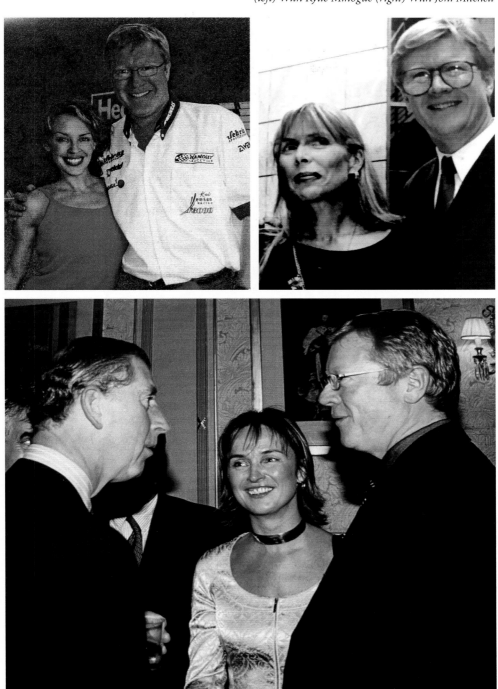

16. I should be so lucky!
(left) With Kylie Minogue (right) With Joni Mitchell

17. Fun at the palace - but not <u>the</u> Palace. Meeting Prince Charles at a Prince's Trust get-together

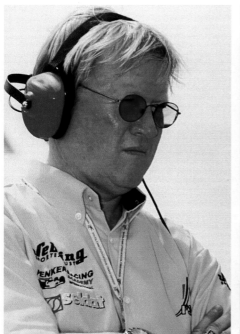

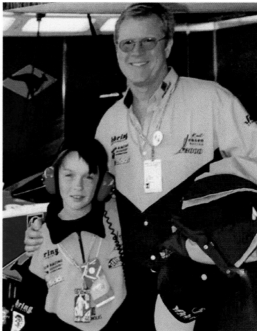

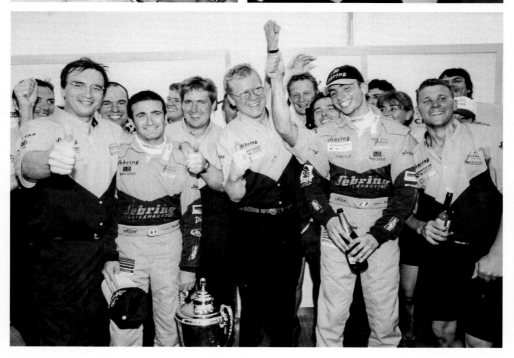

18. Kid Jensen Racing

Top: (left) DJ listening to his drivers out on the track
(right) The Kid and the real Kid, who went on to race in F3
Bottom: The team celebrate their momentus Formula 3000 win at Silverstone, 1999
Courtesy Vincent Franceschini

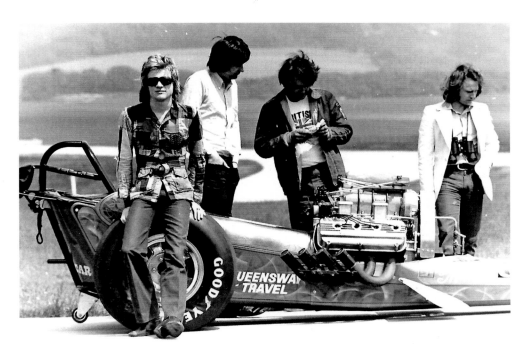

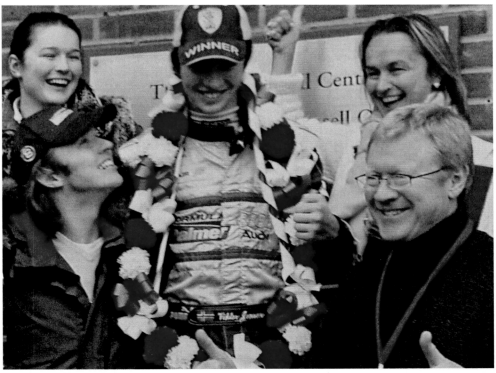

19. Like father, like son
Top: Kid (left) enjoying 208's drag car sponsorship, with Paul Burnett far right. ©Nicole Burnett
Bottom: Viktor Thor takes the plaudits

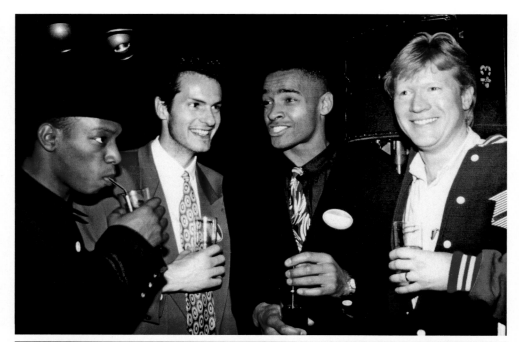

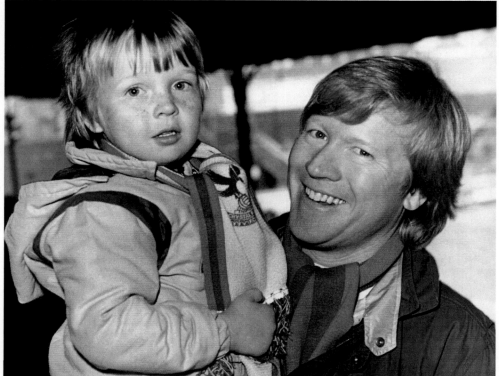

19. Top: Palace pals - with Ian Wright, Dave Madden and Mark Bright celebrating the Eagles' 8-0 win over Southend United in September 1990, in which both Wright and Bright scored a hat-trick

Bottom: 4-year-old Alexander at his first Crystal Palace match ©Hy Money

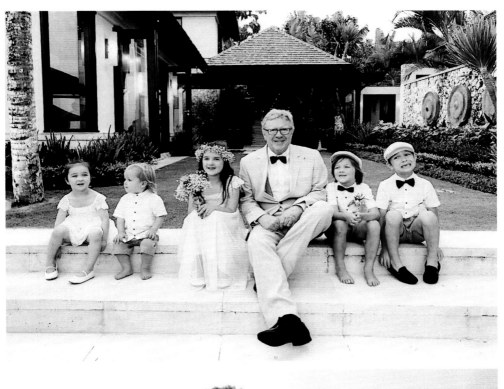

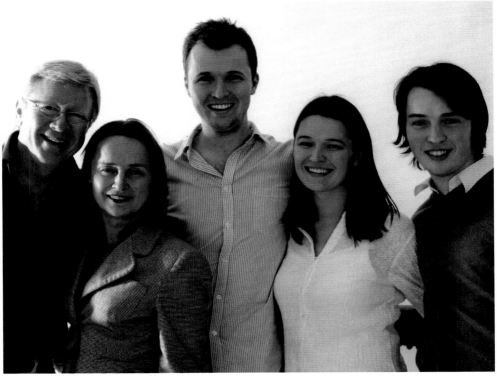

20. Top: With grandchildren in Bali
Bottom: David, Guðrún, Alexander, Anna Lisa and Viktor Thor

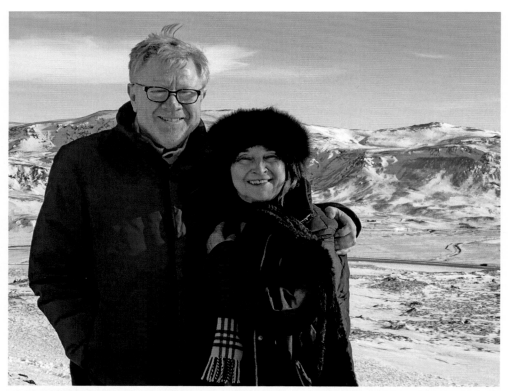

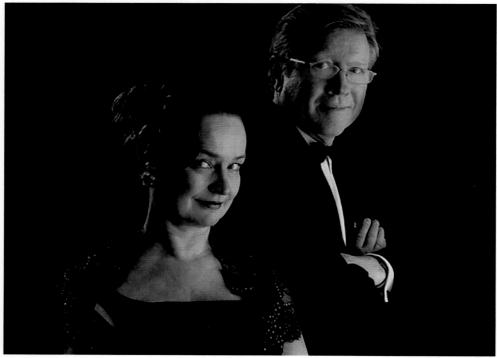

21. Top: David and Guðrún in Iceland, March 2020
Bottom: The name's Jensen... Kid Jensen

14.

LIVING IN AMERICA

Bob Wussler, president of the mighty CBS TV in the US, was in London on business for a few days. Turning on the TV in his hotel room one morning in 1980, he caught the end of an Open University programme on the subject of 'Heroes'. It was hosted by me.

There is a lot of luck in any broadcasting career.

Evidently liking what he saw, my agent took a call from this highly-influential executive, with an address book to die for, inviting me over to the US to become a news anchor in Georgia. Bob was about to leave CBS to join TBS (Turner Broadcasting System), and to co-found the satellite news channel CNN. Everyone knew Bob. Likeable, prematurely grey and a theatrical hugger, his smiley face concealed the toughness and ability which lay below, as required from a man of his stature.

The opportunity appealed to the little boy in me who had grown up watching the grainy TV pictures as former fighter pilot John Glenn became the first American to orbit the Earth in 1962. The chance to work for the guy who helped to produce that historic coverage beamed around the world was unmissable. Having read about his latest idea of the 24-hour news channel, I knew its parent company was where I needed to be. Here was a chance to break out of a music radio pigeonhole and join a company which was making news a rock 'n' roll property.

Increasingly, as I grew older, BBC Radio 4 and LBC had become part of my listening repertoire and I wondered about exploring a more challenging opportunity than my Radio 1 shows of the time. On my Radio Luxembourg programme I had been a newsreader of sorts, but there is a gulf between screaming a few hurried rip-and-read scripts from the *Daily Mirror* punctuated by over-dramatic Morse code effects and delivering a full news programme in-vision to viewers in America, Canada and Hawaii. I also preferred to forget the story in a Luxy bulletin about the Middle East, in which I declared, without realising, that 'lesbian troops' – rather than 'Lebanese troops' – were gathering.

Undeterred, I seized the TBS opportunity in May 1980 and prepared to move from London to a shirt-and-tie job on the other side of the world.

Our belongings were packed up, our beloved Arrow put in quarantine, and we prepared to vacate our much-loved new-build terraced home in Kingston-on-Thames, where our family had truly settled. Warren and Jenny were neighbours we would miss, and the story of our first meeting, with Warren's amazement at our big red telephone when he called around to borrow it before theirs was connected, emerged as a fond tale. They became the sort of supportive and close friends whom we missed from far-off Iceland and Canada, and Warren's passing on in 2013 was to hit us all hard.

The move to Atlanta posed other challenges, with a lively two-year-old and Guðrún's pregnancy. Thankfully, she recognised the scale of the US opportunity for me, and she is a well-travelled free spirit.

Guðrún also connected with Atlanta for peculiar reasons. Her Icelandic mother had mastered English through her overseas travel, and put it to good use by working as a guide on the cruise ships that came to Reykjavík. On one voyage she met Walter Candler, the son of Asa Griggs Candler, who had founded the Coca Cola company in Atlanta. Walter later proposed to her. She was twenty, he was forty. For reasons of distance and the age gap, the offer was not accepted, but the stories of his persistence – and the boxes of apples and oranges he shipped to her family in Iceland – together with the photographs of the family's impressive home in Druid Hills in Atlanta, all became the stuff of family legend.

Despite the attraction and excitement of my move, walking out of Broadcasting House was a wrench. At the time, Radio 1 excelled at caring for its own, with partners and families often thoughtfully invited to relevant station occasions, so it was typical that the secretaries and receptionists convened a lunchtime farewell function for me and Guðrún. I then prepared for a final reflective show, indulging in some of my favourite tracks, with cameo appearances from several of the Radio 1 names of whom I had become fond.

As my last song – 'Surf's Up' from the Beach Boys – faded, I also said goodbye to the name 'Kid', as it was thought to be potentially ill-fitting for the serious content I might have to confront in my grown-up job. 'Kid Jensen was no more,' Paul Gambaccini and I commented on the final handover: 'David Allan Jensen reigns from next week.'

As another chapter ended, I then swapped chairs to become a studio guest, alongside Elton and Frankie Valli, as Paul Gambaccini hosted my *Roundtable*. To this day he has kept a copy of that night's running order, signed by us all.

On settling into my new life in the US, it was touching to later receive generous farewell gifts from both: a case of champagne from Frankie and a crate of Cristal champagne from Elton.

The US channels I was to be part of were owned by the buccaneering Ted Turner, 'The Mouth of the South', a maverick who had inherited his wealth from his father's billboard business – and cut his own hair. He was recognisable instantly from the rear, owing to its crooked angle. He also chose to drive a Toyota Corolla when he could have had a fleet of Cadillacs in his garage. Ted was not a man for meetings, shunning laborious audience research in favour of just popping out of the office to talk to the cab drivers about what they thought of last night's TV. His gift was finding the right people and casting them in the right place. Across the company, I witnessed a 'can-do' culture. If Ted Turner or Bob Wussler liked an idea, they placed their trust in us and ran with it.

One of Ted's pet projects on the channel was a feel-good programme called *Nice People,* which I hosted for a period. Highlighting the endeavours of those who made a difference, from inspiring teachers in rough areas to selfless fundraisers, it reflected his ambition to secure good quality family television rather than yet more comedies. *Nice People* earned an Emmy award nomination, although the programme title was more popular with some people than others. Ted chose it, so I decided to like it too.

The ten o'clock evening news programme was my main presentation role, serving as the centrepiece of the TBS television schedule. Having said that, my arrival on-screen was often delayed in favour of the final stages of an Atlanta Braves baseball game. Turner had bought the team itself because coverage lured viewers, with the added benefit that the money the channel paid out for commentary rights was simply paid into another of his own companies.

The format of my programme was a responsible news magazine, juggling news scripts, interviews and reports. After over a decade in radio, mastering the new art of television news delivery and using the teleprompter was a new experience. It was the first time too I had been supported by a talent coach whilst on-air, who behaved in the way of a football manager geeing up his team at half time. As the cameras cut from me whenever the show moved to a pre-recorded report, Bob Hewitt used to stride across rubbing his hands together, offering encouragement to make sure that I had the right level of energy and the appropriate mood for the next piece.

By coincidence, one of the regular guests on my programme was Coretta, the wife of Martin Luther King – the 'hero' featured on the Open University programme which had earned me the job.

The channel seemed concerned about my voice. This Canadian, they believed, sounded far too English. A voice coach, Lilian Gish, was duly parachuted in from Chicago to sort me out, and help my accent and vocabulary sound more like an all-American dude. I felt in good company when I learned that another client was George HW Bush, the father of George W Bush, who was on the ascendancy when the Reagan-Bush ticket won the 1980 presidential election. I was even treated to filmed examples of Mr Bush senior to illustrate the work she had done.

Marietta in Atlanta had become home, a city connected closely with the Civil War history which had fascinated me at school. TBS looked after me well, and I enjoyed all the trappings of commercial success that a US media career brings, including a house resplendent with antebellum columns and a pool. The latter was the centre of a drama, when a Cottonmouth poisonous snake decided to join my mother for swim. TBS also put two nice cars at our disposal, a perk diminished somewhat by the fact I had yet to learn to drive; a necessity for most Americans. A test was duly arranged, for which I had to meet the examiner some distance away, at a Baptist church in the real hillbilly land of rural Georgia. One of two people enrolled for scrutiny that day, I noted the other person signing their name with a cross. The test seemed to go well, conducted by a large Mrs Doubtfire-type character. At the end she put her clipboard gently down, gave me a huge hug and declared: 'Well, honey – you passed.' This was not England.

The period was memorable for its news agenda, with several key stories developing in my time there, including the Iran hostage crisis which saw a stand-off between the United States and Iran when fifty-two American diplomats and citizens were held hostage for well over a year. I was even scheduled to be despatched to Iran to cover their release, until plans changed.

Ted was a canny operator, and soon sensibly realised that using two separate news services for the two channels was a luxury, when his CNN could provide content for both. It was therefore mooted that I be moved across to CNN to become entertainment producer. The suggestion did not appeal. Talking to Liza Minnelli on the red carpet was not my ambition when I made the long trip across the world; and a hot and humid LA did not seem the best climate in which to bring up our two young children.

One Saturday afternoon, when shuffling my scripts and preparing to deliver a bulletin between the wrestling and baseball on TBS, I heard my name being called. Looking up, I saw the familiar faces of three members of the Police. This was at the height of their World fame, when 'Don't Stand So Close to Me' was topping the charts. 'What are you doing here?' Sting asked, 'You belong in Britain.' The irony of those words from a man living in a New York penthouse was not lost on either of us, but his words struck a chord.

Sting recognised me from BBC Radio 1 where, in Police's early reggae-dominated days, we had recorded a session with them. Its broadcast prompted a surprising two-page letter to me from Sting's mother about how grateful she was, and how much my championing her son's music had meant to the Sumner family.

Another taste of home was a stock report which crept into my news programme about how Dallas had emerged as the world centre for the radio jingle industry. To illustrate how the talents of the city's vocalists were being aired on stations across the world, clips were included of them belting out the familiar Radio 1 melodies, followed by an interview with my old boss Johnny Beerling. Taken aback after seeing the feature in the middle of my own programme, I confessed it seemed a little being 'in the twilight zone'.

The phone rang early one morning. At the other end crackled through a call from London, where it was afternoon, and I heard the familiar tones of Johnny and Paul Burnett. They had been talking about me and decided to say hello and tell me I was missed. I missed them too. Even hearing Gerry Raffety's 'Baker Street' reminded me of a crowded London Tube, and stiffened my resolve to get my agent geared up to engineer a return to my adopted home.

○

In the US, if you liked sport the Monday night football programme on TV was essential viewing, attracting huge audiences. In December 1980, that flagship programme was interrupted. John Lennon had been shot dead outside his Manhattan apartment. The report switched swiftly to New York. as stunned reporters tried to get to grips with what happened when a troubled former security guard carrying a pistol and a paperback copy of *Catcher in the Rye* seized the life of an icon.

Although I had met all his bandmates. I had never managed to meet John, but simply felt the same way that people across the world did that day. The sound of his voice, the power of his lyrics and the gift of his melodies simply epitomised a time and a place in history. Lennon was gone. Any chance of the Beatles ever reuniting was snuffed out, a chapter closed for us all. His death instantly became one of the rare 'where were you when…' moments we each experience in life.

Pausing in heavy traffic in my metallic blue Toyota Celica at an interchange on my way to the studios next day, 'Imagine' echoed from every car as it was played repeatedly on our local station WQXI 'Quixie in Dixie'. With fellow motorists in tears around me, I suddenly felt a long way from home.

A final catalyst for a career move was another timely cameo

from a holidaying Doreen Davies and her husband Derek Mills from the BBC, who had helped to engineer my original journey to Radio 1. When Derek asked jauntily when I would be joining Radio 2, I assured him I would be flattered to when the time was right. Doreen then asked if I was enjoying life in Atlanta, adding pointedly that she had not noticed people looking at me in the streets 'like they do in Britain'. When I mumbled back that public recognition was not my personal career barometer, she responded firmly 'You only have one career.'

Doreen always was a fund of good advice, always offered directly.

As I reflect at my career, I muse whether I left the US too soon. Had the proposed new gig taken me to New York rather than LA, I may have chosen to stay longer. As it was, 1981 saw my return back 'home' to the Radio 1 family; still said to be the most popular station in Britain. Sporting a shorter hair-cut, and now known as David, I was quoted by the *Radio Times* as saying 'My only reservation about coming back is that things happen so quickly. I've had a lot of catching up to do.'

Moving your family across the world is a major job. I glanced at the huge boxes of albums stacked up against the wall in my Atlanta basement, including rarities, early editions and records autographed by the artist, concluding all would be easily replaced if not taken back to London. Such is the naivety of youth: life will go on forever, alongside all the opportunities and privilege it brings. I clearly thought that the likes of Joni Mitchell would autograph something else for me whenever I wanted. In Joni's case, thankfully she did – signing one of her paintings for me in due course – but, as I now recognise, other treasures of an incredible musical era can never be replaced.

The true value of that collection is inestimable, but back then the hefty pile was simply an expensive headache. TBS had originally paid to transport my chattels across to the US, but that generosity did not extend to the shipping back when I returned. As I made plans to rejoin the BBC, I winced at the likely carriage cost to London of my records. Albums are heavier than they look. The only pragmatic solution seemed to be to give away my coveted collection to a good home. Unsurprisingly, a host of eager colleagues from the channel, wide-eyed with amazement, arrived to rummage around in my basement and take away whatever gems took their fancy.

A handful of prized items survived the cull and travelled home with us in our luggage. Who could part with signed albums from Sinatra, Elvis, Lennon and the Stones?

I will not be the last presenter to dispose of their music library in the wrong way at the wrong time. To a DJ, their own music collection is more than a pile of records. Each one is a page in a diary, telling of a time and a place in their life.

15.

NIGHT-TIME RADIO 1

John Peel was knowledgeable, charismatic, and very funny. He had been kind to me in my early innocent days when I knew no-one, and I treasured his friendship enormously. On-air on Radio 1 from its debut weekend in 1967, following a brief yet memorable spell on his late-night *Perfumed Garden* programme on pirate Radio London, he had amassed huge credibility through his music passion, communicated authentically in his deadpan, self-deprecating, erudite bumbling. I, however, still picture us simply as the odd couple hosting *Top of the Pops* together dressed in all manner of random costumes.

In my Luxembourg days, we knew of each other from our rival channels and both took our music seriously, but, as I suggested when speaking to *Deejay* magazine in November 1972, our tastes differed: 'In England I really have to watch out for this... people do say "Jensen, Peel... the same thing!" It's not at all. Just listen to the programmes and you will find this difference in our musical tastes.'

Our first encounter came at a Decca reception in London for Irish singer Fran O'Toole, shortly before Fran and his fellow band members were shot dead in 1975 in one of the most notorious incidents of the Troubles. John and I bonded instantly at the reception, where he told me that he listened to my Luxy programme when journeying home late at night, to the extent that he dubbed the roundabout that he crossed as my programme began as 'Kid Jensen's roundabout'.

John had worked on Radio Luxembourg himself in 1971, hosting an imaginatively offbeat and short-lived programme called *Stenhousemuir 2, Cowdenbeath 2*, a title inspired randomly by the delivery of classified football results. John recorded the show in our London studios, where a self-op turntable arrangement was cobbled together so he could play in his own records, as he had done on the pirate stations.

By the time we were united at Radio 1 our tastes had evolved, with me settling a little more along the pop end of the spectrum than he had. So whilst I played the Police, Toto and Simple Minds, he preferred to cue up Nirvana. We fought for musical supremacy, and when he announced in the office that he was about to play a particular new song, I used to tell him with glee that I had played it the previous week, remaining poker-faced as he tried to detect my level of bluff. We certainly battled for sessions with bands we identified as having future promise, and I claimed the Smiths, Culture Club, Police, Frankie Goes to Hollywood, the Pretenders and the Pet Shop Boys.

This bearded guy from Merseyside, more than a decade older than me, was nakedly emotive. I walked in one day to find him lying on the floor of the hallway just outside the BBC studio, his eyes moist with tears. It transpired that he had been crying for joy after Liverpool had won the European Cup. We hugged and, at his request, I got his show underway until he felt able to steel himself sufficiently to take control.

John arrived early each day at the BBC for his programmes, and he and I enjoyed spending time together, often popping down the road to the Gaylord on Oxford Street for a quick meal. If we had time, he was ever keen to forage in antique shops, on the hunt particularly for ornate Japanese swords to add to his collection.

If we had not caught up before my programme, he would venture into my studio whilst I was on-air, plonking himself across from me at one of the guest mics and chatting to me over the garden fence whilst the tracks played. On one occasion, during a brief exchange on-air he mentioned how much he craved a curry. The terrific Billy Bragg was driving by Portland Place at the time with his then roadie Andy Kershaw and, knowing of the Gaylord's reputation, and loving John, called in to buy a takeaway which he delivered promptly to him at the BBC.

This sort of close partnership and friendship for presenters who followed each other on the schedule was not common. In some cases, the very moment of programme handover was the only contact colleagues had.

John lived in a village called Great Finborough in Suffolk, with his full home address one of those which fills the whole envelope when sending a Christmas card. The University of East Anglia was not too far away, so when I was booked for a gig there he asked if I might allow him to come along. John did few appearances of this ilk, and said he just wanted to come to watch as he felt he had never mastered the art. He made clear he was just accompanying me and did not want a big introduction on the mic. True to his word, he acted as my chauffeur that night and willingly served as my roadie at the end. That was John. As for keeping a low profile, even standing furtively at the back he proved a bigger draw than me amongst the student crowd.

His sardonic sense of humour was renowned, and I watched his conversation in his Radio 1 office in awe as he sparred with long-time producer John Walters. On-air he was hugely entertaining, seemingly just by being himself, but if ever I commented favourably on something I had heard him say he was puzzled, suggesting he wanted to be remembered for the tracks he played not how he 'stumbled into them'. On the contrary, John could play nursery rhymes and still make me want to hang on his every word.

I'm Sorry I Haven't A Clue on Radio 4 was one of his favourite radio programmes, citing its host Humphrey Lyttelton as his best-loved radio presenter. John himself was certainly a more flexible broadcaster than maybe he acknowledged, and his Radio 4 programme *Home Truths* suited his character absolutely, although it puzzled me that some critics suggested that this music anarchist had 'sold out' by hosting a chatty programme about family anecdotes. His whole approach confirmed the adage that everyone has a story in them, and his demeanour was perfect in teasing them out. It was inspired casting.

My own *Home Truths* anecdote might relate to the day I scored at Wembley, but John would have interrupted to remind me that he fed me the ball. He was on the wing, playing in the Radio 1 'celebrity team'. A treasured photograph recorded the moment, with John and I pictured on the pitch with the scoreboard behind us: England 2. Scotland 1.

To be in his company was a privilege and, years after we worked together, he became one of those special, rare friends where you just pick up where you left off, whether days or years apart. We always had something to talk or moan about. I considered myself a hypochondriac, illustrated well when Carly Simon dropped in and we spent more time discussing our cold remedies than music. John was even worse, although his references to health and longevity were a little darker both on and off-air.

'Hello tubs,' said John, pushing two fingers in my stomach. It was to be the last time I saw him. We met at the Yorkshire Grey, a popular Holborn pub with the BBC fraternity. Conversation did turn to health, as it tends to with people of a certain age, and he spoke of his diabetes, showing off the insulin pens he was required to use. He was cheered by an article he had read trumpeting the benefits to the heart of the antioxidants present in red wine, but then became dismayed on calculating just how many cases he would have to drink to bring any appreciable value.

The news of his death in 2004, aged just 65, stunned me. He and Sheila, the wife to whom he referred as 'The Pig' owing to the way she snorted when laughing, were on holiday in Peru when he suffered a sudden heart attack in his hotel room. By then, I was working on Capital Radio hosting the morning show and was devastated to be called by a BBC journalist for a tribute quote. There is no good way to hear news like that, but that certainly was not the best. The story was to make the front page of the majority of the British press, from the *Times* and the *Telegraph* to the *Sun* and the *Daily Express*. The first record played after his death was announced on Radio 1's *Newsbeat* was his anthem, the Undertones' 'Teenage Kicks'.

John Peel was a droll guy who lit up a room. People gravitated to him, and regarded him as a guru, with many huge names feeling indebted to his having identified their early promise. Despite that huge regard, he was a thoroughly ordinary person who chose to run his own affairs rather than surround himself with an entourage or the BBC's machine. He never acknowledged that he was a star – but he was. I miss him.

My return to Radio 1 appeared, in time, to be worthy of a mention in the BBC's august *Annual Report and Handbook* for 1983. Initially, I was at the helm of a music and talk programme called *Studio B15*, produced by Radio 4 and named imaginatively after the studio from where it originated, before being appointed to the Radio 1 evening show which aired just before Peel's late-night shindiggery. Our programmes delivered the more serious and fresher end of Radio 1's musical offering, supplying an invaluable alibi to the BBC hierarchy when pestered for evidence of Radio 1's distinctiveness. I was certainly permitted more musical freedom to play what I felt to be appropriate than I had been on the earlier programme. John referred to our shows as a 'steam valve' for the network, letting off pressure from a music press critical of the convenience food served up during daytime. We were referred to collectively as 'Night-time Radio 1', and I dubbed us 'the Rhythm Pals'.

The premier pairing of John Walters and John Peel lodged in an office on the third floor of Egton House, the floor down from the daytime programmes. Heaving with white tape boxes containing spools of session recordings, John sat on piles of old records because there was only room for one chair. Rumour has it that one production office had not been entered by a cleaner since 1967.

My producer Mike Hawkes and I lodged in the small office next door, from where he usually based himself whilst our evening programme was on-air, particularly if there were guests to shepherd to the studio. The voyage between the two was lengthy and spooky in the night-time hours after the reception area had closed, necessitating catching the lift to the basement before climbing down some steps, switching on the light and walking into a tunnel which ran under the road and shook to the noise of the Bakerloo Line, before emerging behind the old reception desk at Broadcasting House and climbing the stairs up to the studios.

Our office served as the venue for meetings with record label representatives eager to secure airplay for their product, which explains why, on one occasion, we turned up to discover Elton John sitting in my chair, poised to give us the heads up about the latest news from his own record company, Rocket Records. Formed with Bernie Taupin, the label handled the likes of Kiki Dee, Randy Edelman and Colin Blunstone, and was no idle hobby. It was clear how serious Elton was about his business and, knowing it so well from all perspectives, he was an excellent plugger.

Friendly rivalry meant John and I competed for the best live sessions. They played a key part in my Radio 1 programmes – and helped to ameliorate the needle-time predicament which, for years, restricted the amount of recorded music UK radio stations could play.

One such session featured Frankie Goes to Hollywood,

prompting a call from Malcolm Geary just afterwards, securing exposure for the band on the Tyne Tees TV music show *The Tube*, after which Trevor Horn got in touch regarding a deal with his record company ZTT. When your gut tells you that you are hearing something special, it is a privilege to be able to play a small part in the careers of talented musicians and, without wishing to sound arrogant, there is a warm feeling of quiet reflected glory when their fortunes rise.

For the sake of completeness, I should mention that there are many bands who did not rise to success despite my best efforts. I fear also that my well-intentioned advice could be thoroughly flawed, for example when Robert Smith shared his plans with me for the Cure. Chatting after a performance at Hammersmith Palais where he was acting as guitarist with Siouxsie and the Banshees, who had already built an impressive reputation, I asked him which direction he was planning to take of the two bands. When he told me his inclination was to focus on his work with the Cure, I drew a sharp intake of breath and suggested he think again in view of the status of Siouxsie and the Banshees, with their great musicians and writers. The Cure were to become an internationally famous act in which he plays a part to this day

In July 1983, the programme featured a session with the Smiths, recordings of which were to appear on the album *Hatful of Hollow*. These were the earliest days of this anti-establishment act, and I was the first person to interview Morrissey: 'First thing we've gotta do is establish for people who may not know anything about you – which I guess is quite a few people outside Manchester – how you came to be in a band called the Smiths.'

As I anticipated from all I knew, this 20-year old was serious about his music, and deep about most things. The trademark gladioli in the back pocket of his jeans whilst he was on stage meant something. Morrissey thought carefully about his answers, speaking about meeting Johnny Marr at a Patti Smith gig and about why he preferred his deal with Rough Trade records rather than one with a major label. In an angle which has not dated too well, we also discussed why 'Manchester had not thrown up the number of bands that Liverpool has'. He suggested that he had little kinship with the city and that he would 'leave very soon' – when he 'became rich'. He now lives in LA.

On long family drives, Smiths tracks are cranked up loudly in our car, with my sons inheriting my love for the lyrical and musical strength of their work. I gather Morrissey has said that a lot of people claim to have been responsible for bringing their music to a wider audience, but flatteringly credits me as a key mover in those early days. He remarked in his autobiography that every time John Peel or I played 'Hand in Glove', 'I stand by the radio listening – a disfigured beast finally unchained from the ocean floor. The song rises out the radio and there is immediate support from music writers of integrity.'[16]

Music interviews featured more heavily on the evening programme than they had on the drive-time show and I relished conducting them, particularly when the artists genuinely opened up about their lives.

Debbie Harry's hair changed colour in the course of one day I spent with her, from blonde to brown. She and her Blondie colleague – and then partner – Chris Stein told me they were taken aback by the enthusiasm of British fans, suggesting the level of acclaim was greater here than anywhere else in the world. Her image became a symbol of the age, lionised as one of the great female icons and one of the most photographed women in the Eighties. In some ways, however, her amazing image as a significant star of post-punk became the focus rather than her amazing voice. Her true gift was illustrated beautifully when talk presenter James Whale and I flew to Monte Carlo for a Fashion

16 *Autobiography*, Morrissey.

Rocks event, and witnessed a breathtakingly pure performance from her, alongside José Carreras.

Hopes were high for a seventh Number One when I spoke to the members of Blondie on Radio 1 in 1984 at the time their book *Making Tracks* was published. Conversation ranged from Dr. Feelgood and Wilko's influence on US music to chat about Debbie giving away her pet rabbit to Central Park zoo when it grew too large and began jumping off the roof. She explained her attention was devoted subsequently to a tank of sea horses.

As one track played, Debbie looked up and asked me what I had left to achieve in my career, with my Radio 1 and TV profile seemingly well in-hand. 'You've got it all,' she said. It was a typically generous and humble comment from someone blessed with her track record, delivered with self-evidently no envy. Such remarks make you pause for thought. One rarely looks at one's own life the way others do, but one blessing of age and reflection is how it helps you appreciate belatedly just how good the good times were.

Artists often surprise. A Hollywood hotel room was the setting for an interview with Little Richard as part of the promotion for his comeback faith-based album *Lifetime Friend*. This colourful character opened the door in full costume, wearing a sparkly suit, cravat and mascara, exclaiming 'My oh my! What have we here? Who have they sent to butter my buns?' before kissing me sloppily mouth-to-mouth. It is not a quote I easily forget.

Sitting by the sea under the Copacabana sun in Rio, Pina Colada in hand, while chatting to Carlos Santana, ranks as the most enjoyable setting for an interview I have ever experienced. If that counts as work, my job is a blessing. I was invited over there to be part of Rock in Rio, one of the largest music festivals in the world, with over 1.5 million people gathering to watch some of the world's biggest music names. I love Brazil, although it tends to be one of those countries where everybody seems to wear a uniform of some sort, and, sadly, poverty greets you around the corner. One highlight of the fashionable Ipanema beach, also in the south zone of the City, is the former Veloso bar where composer Tom Jobim and poet Vinícius de Moraes saw the girl who passed by in the winter of 1962 and inspired the song 'Garota de Ipanema' – 'The Girl From Ipanema'.

The Stranglers were rarely out the news for a spell, claiming to be banned not only by venues but by whole countries following the role they played in disrupting the Seventies. Their then frontman Hugh Cornwell visited Radio 1 for an extended interview in 1983, around the time of the release of their album *Feline* and immediately prior to their appearance on *Top of the Pops*.

Despite this being an age of postage stamps rather than the convenience of email, a huge volume of correspondence was received from patient listeners hoping that I might make use of the questions they had suggested for my Stranglers encounter. Hugh seemed a little wary about the topics that might arise, but I relied on the old trick of distracting him with an initial warm-up question unrelated to his music.

As always with Hugh, the conversation was both fascinating and earnest, focusing at first on their bleak image. His response cited a fascinating short documentary he and bandmate Jet Black had researched and produced for BBC West in 1982 called *The Colour Black*. The programme, featuring the views of academics in corduroy jackets, asserted the colour was often a symbol of authority, as demonstrated by the vestments of religious figures or the police. Hugh suggested the band had adopted it because it was not on the spectrum, allowing people to infer what they wished from their music rather than from a manufactured image. Paradoxically, their blank canvas cultivated an image so colourful, it is recalled with ease to this day.

As he left the studio, Hugh was given all the letters for reference or reply, and he had been keen during the interview to repeatedly give out an address for the band. In an era when radio was less interactive than nowadays, and when music stars did not cultivate the direct ongoing dialogue with listeners they now do via social media, Hugh's level of fan engagement seemed ahead of its time.

To meet your heroes is often a dangerous thing. All the colourful traits which help build a truly creative artist their reputation are the very ones which risk making an encounter disappointing… and sometimes the fault was mine.

Having hankered after spending some time with Van Morrison, I was delighted to learn that the gifted musician had asked specifically for me to carry out an interview. But with his reputation for being 'difficult', 'touchy' and reluctant to talk about music, little wonder I was trembling as I climbed unaccompanied into the lift at the Royal Lancaster Hotel.

Major artists are often accompanied by an unwieldy entourage of lieutenants: any, or all, of the record company, manager, PR team and minders. But on this occasion, as Van the Man greeted a nervous me at the door, he did not look too much like a star – and he was alone.

I tried. I tried so hard to get the best from him and to make the interview as good as it possibly could be, but every careful question I posed was met by a pause and a gruff ten second answer. The longer he took to answer, the more I tried to fill the embarrassing gaps, flustering around trying to improve my question and make the answering easier. I perched myself on one bed in his twin room. He sat opposite on the other and I swung the microphone between us. Then, he rose and moved across to sit on the only chair in the room. I followed with my microphone and bulky Uher reel-to-reel tape recorder, supposedly portable but very heavy, and stooped down beside him, trying to persist with the questioning.

Up he got again. This time, moving towards his bed – where, this time, he decided to lie. I kneeled on the floor by his duvet, and again attempted to continue posing deep, probing questions about his art. Then he turned over on the bed to face the wall. It was a farcical sight. I eventually said something like 'We're not getting far here', made my excuses and hurriedly left, mic lead dangling.

In the foyer, other victims awaited their turn and I volunteered an honest yet tactful assessment of my encounter with the man we all regarded so highly. At the time, I concluded that he was just being 'assey' that day but, on reflection, I was simply being too impatient. A golden interview rule is you should always afford the interviewee time and space to answer, rather than jumping in. I also learned that Van has to know someone quite well before he opens up, and in my nervousness and keenness not to take up too much of his time, I had not even tried to form an elementary bond before launching into my interrogation.

Van was looked after by Scottish songwriter Bill Martin, a hugely accomplished figure who had penned some of the biggest hits for the Bay City Rollers, Cilla Black and Slik, as well as 'Congratulations' for Cliff and 'Puppet on a String' for Sandie Shaw. After the interview, Bill phoned me at home to establish whether the interview had been fruitful. I was honest. 'Not great, Bill. My questions outweighed his answers. There were gaps. It's going to take a lot of editing. It's not going to sound good.' Concerned for his client's reputation, and keen to do me proud as a champion of Van's music, he undertook to see what he could do.

A couple of years later, when I bumped into him again, he enquired if Van had been in touch to arrange a second interview, as he had said he would. No, I said. I have been waiting for that call ever since.

Bill died in March 2020, not long after I attended his 80th birthday party at the Caledonian Club in Belgravia. The funeral of Bill Martin MBE was sadly one of those confined to few attendees owing to the precautions introduced to tackle Covid-19.

I did meet Van subsequently, and still respect him hugely. You cannot listen to his work or see him on stage and not do so. Known as a hard taskmaster and utter perfectionist, he sings from the soul with an enviable dynamic range, and the construction of his songs was way ahead of its time. Like me, his father was a jazz enthusiast and he had grown up in Belfast steeped in the jazz age, developing a love and respect for the beauty of American jazz. Yet still he was the master of his own music.

My most touching encounter with Van had come years before, in my Luxembourg days, when his second album *Astral Weeks* was released in 1968. It was getting talked about in all the music press, with much attention in *Rolling Stone*. A radical departure from his earlier pop hits, it was highly impressive, particularly considering he had been little more than a teenager when he wrote the songs. I played the whole of one side of the album on-air on Radio Luxembourg, then flipped it over and played the other. Surprised colleagues hurried down to the studio to see me, asking what the album was, and were impressed with what I had dared to do.

Shortly afterwards, a letter arrived from Van's American wife, whose memorable name was Janet Planet. She wrote that she and Van had been driving through Holland when I had played it, and told how much they had enjoyed hearing it in its entirety on their car radio. Just as with Bill Wyman mentioning in his memoir that the Stones tuned in to me on their tour bus, one of the many beauties of radio is you never know who is listening.

Van went on to mention Radio Luxembourg on his *Englightenment* album in the lyrics to the track 'In the Days Before Rock 'N' Roll', on which he collaborated with the Irish poet Paul Durcan.

'We went over the wavebands (ssss... sssss)
We'd get Luxembourg
Luxembourg and Athlone'

16.

TOP OF THE POPS

As I pushed open the door of my *Top of the Pops* dressing room in February 1978, it appeared that I was not to benefit from its exclusive use. A lacy black dress dangled from the hook on the wall. It belonged, I was informed, to Kate Bush. A hasty informal rota for the room preserved modesty as we prepared for our appearances.

'And now, making her debut on *Top of the Pops* is the exquisite Kate Bush, with her new single, 'Wuthering Heights'.'

Aged 20 and seemingly without nerves, she crouched by the piano on stage, pumping out the now-familiar bewitching melody. Such was the distinctiveness of both her appearance and the song that she awoke next day as a celebrity, going on to become the first female to top the UK charts with a self-composed song. *Top of the Pops* had that power.

The programme had begun on New Year's Day in 1964, and by its Seventies' heyday it was attracting around fifteen million viewers each week, emerging as a defining BBC TV show. It is difficult now to comprehend just how influential this Thursday night ritual was. Whilst daytime Radio 1 was often criticised by sharp-tongued music press critics and the cool and hip gang around town for being too mainstream, there was something about the heritage and scale of *Top of the Pops* which meant it was excused and still lauded, even if it did feature Terry Wogan's 'Floral Dance' or 'There's No-one Quite Like Grandma' by the St Winifred's School Choir. It was a family show, and I became part of its rich history in 1977.

The programme was filmed on Thursdays in Studio 4 at the iconic TV Centre in West London, with its familiar circular glass entrance. Fan clubs pooled information about the identities of the week's artists and the entrance that each might use, so that their followers could catch a glimpse of their heroes; and the record labels also did their best to fuel the hubbub to ensure the loudest cheers for their acts.

After a change in the rules in 1966, miming to recorded tracks was not allowed and music was supposed to be played live under Musicians' Union rules. Artists who had spent weeks agonising in the studio to ensure perfection for a track thus had to be content with a live accompaniment from the session musicians and backing singers on the set. Although the house band comprised gifted individuals, they were only afforded a couple of hours to rehearse all the required tracks, and were also probably more familiar with orchestrations from a previous generation than Seventies pop and rock hits. Manchester outfit New Order was the only one I recall playing completely live, although there were serious sound problems on that occasion and the exercise was not repeated in my time.

Bob Marley arrived with his sizeable entourage. Although a laid-back guy who said little, he had a real aura and was the most compelling and charismatic performer I ever witnessed live on my time on the show. Determined to play his guitar in the studio on 'Satisfy My Soul', the rhythm section was so intricate it gave me chills down my spine.

The producer in my early days was Robin Nash, a bow-tie wearing theatrical fellow with a wonderful sense of humour. He was disarmed, however, when the Damned turned up for the camera check. The band's Captain Sensible, now known for his trademark red beret, appeared instead in a full wedding dress. Robin refused to let him appear unless he changed.

Michael Hurll succeeded Robin. Michael was the prolific light entertainment producer who worked with Cilla Black and Cliff Richard, and was executive producer of *The Two Ronnies*. Amongst the ideas Michael hatched was to send us occasionally to other countries to host the show and reflect their biggest hits. John Peel journeyed to Amsterdam, and I was despatched to Singapore, only to discover that an equivalent chart there did not seem to exist. The concept was short-lived.

Under Hurll's direction, about a hundred eager young fans hurried through the door each week, wearing progressively more colourful Day-Glo clothes to the extent that the occasion began to resemble a New Year's Eve party. His strategy was to make the audience part of the performance, with the aid of flags and hats – and cheerleaders to whip up the energy.

Seeking to play my part in fuelling the excitement, I sometimes involved nearby onlookers in my on-screen chat between songs. That impromptu tactic played poorly just before one performance. 'Hot Chocolate next,' I announced, before turning to a girl just over my shoulder and adding, 'You look like you like them a lot.' 'I can't stand them,' she retorted. Frontman Errol Brown wisely just turned away.

Gordon Elsbury, Michael Hurll's right-hand man, was a lovely, funny and obliging guy. An energetic coach, he conducted proceedings on the floor with a flourish, waving his arms, pointing, and generally making sure that all those involved in the show looked as they should in order to create the necessary mood, and get the best from you.

It was in the gift of the *Top of the Pops* producer to determine which Radio 1 presenters would host the show but, surprisingly, *not* commonplace for presenters to naturally plug their programme during their appearance. Michael Hurll worshipped John Peel, restoring him to the rota after earlier nervous disappointments. He seemed fond too of the Peel-Jensen double act, which we preferred to execute live rather than pre-record, despite John's daring wry introductions which particularly chimed with the cameramen and directors' sense of humour: 'The guys who put the big into country, Big Country…'; 'Here come the rock'n'roll accountants – Toto…'; and David Grant, 'dressed in what appears to be a fire hydrant.' One more barbed remark referred to Queen's performances at the Sun City Super Bowl in Bophuthatswana, South Africa, at the time of apartheid when the Musicians' Union had advised that artists should not visit. Although John was not forgiven by Queen for some time, he seemed undaunted.

When working as a pair, John and I shared a dressing room and after being given the keys and getting settled we used to walk across to the sound booth to pre-record the chart rundown before being briefed on the programme itinerary in a café by one of Gordon's clipboard-carrying helpers.

This was the era when *Top of the Pops* was beginning to feel sufficiently confident to poke fun at itself, so next stop was the wardrobe department, given our penchant for wearing all manner of costumes on dubious pretexts. John and I dressed as footballers, the Blues Brothers and Robin Hood and his Merry Man. On one occasion, when we requested something on a Roman theme we returned to our dressing room to find two sheets hanging from hooks on the wall, and the instruction from giggling costume staff to fashion a toga with them.

Puncturing an urban myth is not a popular pursuit, but I should offer my account of a performance that has gone down in history, when Dexys Midnight Runners appeared in 1982 on a special *Top of the Pops* edition marking Radio 1's fifteenth anniversary.

The band was set to perform their cover of Van Morrison's 'Jackie Wilson Said (I'm in Heaven When You Smile)'. During rehearsal, I noticed that a photograph of the darts player Jocky Wilson was being used as a backdrop rather than that of American soul artist Jackie Wilson. I quickly informed the floor manager, who grabbed his walkie-talkie to alert colleagues and darted away, I presumed to rectify matters. The show, however, was aired with Jocky's picture still in view.

Several commentators mentioned the matter in disbelief over the ensuing days, not least some fellow Radio 1 presenters on-air. Dexys' Kevin Rowland, however, later claimed that the errant picture had been a deliberate ploy to remind people that they had a sense of humour having earned a reputation as taking themselves too seriously. Kevin later told the *Guardian* that they had instructed the wrong picture be used 'For a laugh', believing that 'only an idiot' would think it was an error.

Regardless, the story of it being a genuine mistake persists to this day... maybe because it is simply a better story.

John Peel had picked up on a 1978 single called 'Jilted John', originally released as a B-side and recorded for just £200. It was written and performed by Jilted John, aka Graham Fellows, during his first term as a drama student at Manchester Polytechnic School of Theatre. John Peel suggested that it had hit potential were it to be picked up by a major label, which EMI did. As I introduced this brutal account of disposable teenage love on *Top of The Pops*, I called it 'One of the most bizarre singles of the decade,' which it was. With the hook bearing the words 'Gordon is a moron', it is interesting that the forename never appears to have made a comeback.

It is reported that *Top of the Pops* was the programme that led two of the Bee Gees to the girls they would marry. The brothers' first appearance was in 1967, and through decades of changing fashions and musical styles, their falsetto tight harmonies ruled, producing twenty albums and selling more than 220 million records worldwide.

Guðrún adored their music, and the brothers got to know us well enough to regularly send us a generous crystal glass gift at Christmas. At one stage, Maurice lived close to us, and I recall a bizarre conversation about refuse collection as we shared the same bin collector round. Maurice told me that the famous drum sound on the front of 'You Win Again' was conceived in his garage with the aid of the bins.

Wearing a fetching tank-top, I introduced the youngest of the Bee Gees, Andy Gibb, on the show in June 1977. Andy was to die tragically young, around a decade later, aged just 30. His brother Maurice passed away in 2003 at the age of 53, and Maurice's twin Robin died in 2012. At Robin's funeral I sat alongside his mother Barbara and the group's manager Robert Stigwood, as we watched remaining brother Barry speak from the heart and offer a fulsome tribute. As we and the other guests slowly filed out the private service in Henley, we shook hands and I told him how touching his words had been. Barry confided that Robin had always been the glue that bound the guys together through all the ups and downs that brothers have, and insisted how important it was always to part on good terms. Barbara was to live to see the deaths of three of her five children.

The edition of *Top of the Pops* aired on Christmas Day 1979 featured the Bee Gees song 'Tragedy', although the group was not seen on screen, with viewers instead feasted to the sight of menacing-looking dancers dressed in silver clown outfits, with their faces whitened. In the days before pop videos, any artist not represented in person on *Top of the Pops* had their record played, accompanied by a fitting lively routine from a troupe of energetic dancers. The most famous distracting entourage was the all-girl Pan's People, choreographed by Flick Colby, clapping and wriggling in their fluorescent costumes. They were replaced briefly in 1976 by the mixed group Ruby Flipper, returning to the all-girl Legs & Co. as the music turned to disco and punk. Some dancers were common to several of the groups, and I still bump into the famous Babs Lord, known for her long blonde hair, who married the actor Robert Powell. Such was the profile of the programme, even the names of the dancers were known by the audiences.

Pan's People arrived in the studio in the morning, well before anyone else, to rehearse their disciplined moves. Although a puzzling sight to today's generation as they stumble across the old shows on TV, the colourful aerobics were a key part of the character of the show. That was confirmed to me on one occasion when I was invited to join a BA pilot in his cockpit on a journey to the US. Shaking my hand, he confessed that seeing their performance was the highlight of his week.

After *Top of the Pops* had been recorded or broadcast, many of the participants wound down in the Green Room, the area reserved traditionally in a theatre or similar venue for performers to linger before and after a performance. On one occasion I walked in to see the familiar huddles of people gathering round each of the artists, but one performer stood alone and ignored. I recognised him as Neil Diamond. I was incredulous that this hugely-gifted tunesmith, whose presence was lauded in Canada and America, seemed barely to attract a second glance in London that day. Nevertheless, it was a great opportunity to introduce ourselves and an unexpected chance for me to enjoy half an hour of quality conversation with one of the best-selling musicians of all time, known not only for performing 'Sweet Caroline', 'Song Song Blue' and 'Cracklin' Rosie', but for a legacy of irreplaceable melodies like 'Red Red Wine'.

Such was the might of both Radio 1 and *Top of the Pops* that the DJs as well as the music performers were regarded as stars. As new names joined Radio 1, even their debut TV appearance was sufficient to boost their equity overnight. Without doubt, this was the show that made me, as recognition is an essential part of what we do.

It can also be flattering, but never more so than on the day I returned to Nottingham to see some friends. Having jumped in a cab at the railway station, I was driven to my old stomping ground on the outskirts of the city in Ruddington. On arrival, the stroll to the pub where we had planned to meet took me past all the shops I remembered from a decade before, still selling the same things and still staffed by the same village characters. They called out to me: 'Welcome back, Kid.' 'Glad you haven't forgotten us.' 'We saw you on *Top of the Pops!*' As they popped out of their shops into the street one-by-one to greet me in what seemed like a scene from *The Sound of Music*, I felt like one of their family being welcomed home.

Radio stations change and, in some ways, they must, with presenters and styles falling in and out of favour. But when John Peel and I heard the rumour in 1984 that our Radio 1 programme timings were to be flipped, with my show in danger of becoming a late-night country show and his being shunted to midnight, we both felt that our counter-culture was at an end and it might be time to consider moving on.

By serendipity, London's Capital Radio got in touch. Tony Hale, the station's head of music with whom I had worked previously on the Radio 1 roadshow and other programmes out of Manchester such as *Quiz Kid,* suggested I should join them, with the bait that I would also host a new chart to be broadcast across all commercial radio stations. The time seemed right to make a move.

Such transfers are often uncomfortable. In a sense, it is your agent's job to choreograph the move, yet you feel you have broken a direct personal loyalty with supportive bosses whom you respect and have got on well with. The prospect of a national chart show was the career reason for being seduced, but, emotionally, I genuinely felt that Capital was closer to the radio I wanted to hear at the time, and it connected with London as no other media did.

Capital thwarted the efforts from my buddy John Peel to join me, as I gather the station did not wish to be regarded as a refuge for disillusioned Radio 1 staff. Long term for him that was a lucky escape, given he was retained by the BBC for a further twenty years until his death, whilst who knows what fate he might have met in commercial radio. John once observed that he received loyalty payments from the BBC, 'But then I think it dawned on them that no-one wanted to seduce me.'[17] My move to Euston Tower was thus a sorrowful separation – one which John wryly suggested amounted to divorce.

I did not stay to grow old at Radio 1, although I was delighted to play a cameo role in *Smashie and Nicey: The End of an Era* in 1994. The one-off BBC TV special built on the success of the Smashie and Nicey characters in *Harry Enfield's Television Programme*, played by Harry Enfield and Paul Whitehouse, parodying ageing celebrity BBC Radio 1 presenters. The station's alumni took it in good spirits, even competing for having inspired elements of the script or performance. Tony Blackburn, Alan Freeman, John Peel and I certainly saw it as a badge of honour to be invited to play ourselves in the special edition. In its opening sequence, Smashie and Nicey were bounding up a corridor in the old Broadcasting House when they bumped into me on the staircase, screaming 'Not now, Kid Pension!' and landing a fierce right-hander which caused me to roll down the stairs. I confess a stunt double executed that final shot, although watching it even deceives me.

Being lampooned is a measure of one's profile, so it was good to be portrayed briefly on *Spitting Image* too. I suspect Fluck and Law laboured less over my puppet than Margaret Thatcher's, relying just on a shock of blond hair and a topical reference to my leaving Radio 1 to do its job.

---

17 *John Peel*, Mick Wall .

A CAPITAL MOVE

Suave Michael Aspel was a familiar sight on TV, hosting programmes such as *Ask Aspel*, *Crackerjack!* and *Give Us A Clue*, before clutching his Big Red Book on *This is Your Life*. He was also an unassailable Capital Radio mainstay, hosting a warm mid-morning music and chat show in London for ten years – and my job in 1984 was to replace this treasure.

I was in good company. By the Eighties, Capital had developed a sound and pace I envied, with a hugely diverse range of presenters each identifying their own territory, from Mick Brown's soul to Nicky Horne, Richard Allinson, Greg Edwards, Tim Westwood's rap show and David Roddigan's excellent Saturday night dub-classics.

Roger Scott reigned. He was a true 'disc jockey' as opposed to 'presenter', truly riding the songs like the most able of equestrians. With enviable energy, pace and polish, his delivery was disciplined and tight, creating a sense of urgency. Roger had the knack of making you feel he was taking you to a destination with a real sense of occasion, whether with his *Three O'Clock Thrill* or his Friday *Cruising*, or simply just the next song. He was to die aged just 46, in 1989 but remains an inspiration for some of the UK's top music presenters.

On the programme schedule, Capital's hour-long evening news programme *The Way It Is* preceded the return of *Anna and the Doc*, when the legendary Anna Raeburn dealt 'frankly with your personal, emotional and sexual problems,' before Mike Dickin took 'your calls on a wide variety of topics.'

This variegated approach to radio would be anathema to today's focused stations, but UK radio at that stage was still catching up and the paucity of few stations meant a less competitive radio market. You could try to be all things to all people, and its earliest catchy jingles from Blue Mink, David Dundas and the London Symphony Orchestra had served to unite the brand and help it to own its city: 'Isn't it good to know Capital Radio.'

Capital's home, Euston Tower, was a landmark; a tower block built in 1970 which loomed over the north side of Euston Road, dubbed 'the Tower of Power' by Everett. Such was radio's prestige and perceived scale, people presumed we occupied all its thirty-six stories, whereas most of the operation was housed on but a single floor. As listeners entered its reception, they were greeted by the receptionist's friendly banter as they gazed across at the iconic spiral staircase which they presumed led to all the layers of showbiz magic above.

On the Capital floor lay the offices and the area dubbed 'the Playpen', where we noisy toddlers congregated before and after our programmes. The studios were typical of their vintage, equipped with reel-to-reel tape machines, turntables and numerous cartridge tape player slots for the ads or jingles. Some changes had been introduced since the station had launched, not least losing the grand piano from the large studio. This had been used to perform music to record for airplay, given stations had been allowed only to play a total of nine hours of records each day and were required contractually to devote at least three percent of net income to the employment of musicians.

When we saw a green Rolls Royce parked illegally just outside the front door, we knew Dickie was in the house. Richard Attenborough was the chairman of Capital Radio, then a proud London company owning a single station. His voice had launched that station in 1973, with 'For the very first time. This is Capital

Radio.'

Theatrical Dickie understood how presenters felt when 'on stage', and always troubled to stop by the studio to say a cheery hello to whoever was on-air. One morning, I was halfway through a show, sporting a Crystal Palace top, when he called in. He paused in the doorway as he caught sight of me, before turning up his nose and incredulously spitting out the words 'Crystal Palace', at which the lifelong Chelsea supporter and later board member promptly turned and walked out again. It was a privilege to be there during the involvement of this award-winning actor, director and producer.

The Attenborough culture permeated the building in the early days. The company cared for its team, even to the extent of staging Christmas parties for the 'Capital kids' – the children of the employees – held against the backdrop of that famous staircase.

The glittering circle of Richard's friends meant that a host of familiar figures were involved in those early days, including Cathy McGowan from TV's influential music show *Ready Steady Go!* and Joanna Lumley, who often called in to Euston Tower. I picture her smiling, oozing all the presence you would expect, poking her head round the studio door asking if I minded her popping in. Who would?

Nigel Walmsley was managing director, a politically-skilled heavyweight figure and former marketing director at the Post Office. Whilst at Capital, he played a key role in establishing RAJAR, a solid audience research currency for UK radio which brought together listening figures to BBC and commercial radio for the first time.

Nigel had appointed Jo Sandilands, a former editor of *Honey* magazine, to the post of programme controller. Some people unfairly suggested her lack of direct radio experience disqualified her from understanding radio. It did not. I found her professional and her thinking solid, although I was intrigued to learn that I was part of their strategy of attracting 'white van man' through playing more male-oriented rock. They felt there were quite sufficient affluent Londoners listening to Lulu, and Gerald Harper playing Bert Kaempfert on Sundays; my role was to complement that audience.

Jo's ambition was to make the station 'spikier', and she volunteered the idea of inviting Julie Burchill on my morning programme regularly, creating a colourful 'appointment to listen'. Julie was a firebrand provocative journalist who had first made her name aged 17 at the *New Musical Express*, gearing up subsequently to pen fiery columns for the national press. In a later column in the *Financial Times* she proclaimed of her notoriety: 'Mr Murdoch's not paying me to sit around to say, "Well, on the other hand." I'm like a fireman: I have a specific job to do and then get out.'

As Jo was a huge fan, she asked me to lure Julie to a lunch. The courtship was fruitful, and I delivered her back to the station to introduce her to Jo, who just looked up in disbelief that I had managed to lasso her idol. Julie's debut broadcast brought forth her convictions on why pretty blondes are popular in Hollywood. The phones rang off the hook, with listeners stirred to respond with equivalent energies and even less restraint. Julie never appeared again.

Graham Dene hosted the Capital Breakfast Show, with his chirpy early morning voice. In an industry famed for rumours and gossips he is one of the nicest guys I know, with not a malicious bone in his body. Walking into his studio one morning I saw him behind the controls as usual, slipping off his headphones, but as I glanced to my left, I caught sight of a smiling visitor sitting opposite. It was the face of the most photographed woman in the world.

Princess Diana was a long-standing fan of Graham's, and she had asked to pay a low-key visit to sit in on his show. Graham gestured for me to sit down whilst he prepared to go live, with just the instruction 'Don't say anything about the Princess.' The guest seats in the Capital studio were a tight fit, so Diana and I spent an uncomfortable few moments before the record ended perched thigh-by-thigh, as I struggled to dream up appropriate Royal small talk. Her favourite song was then played – Billy Joel's 'Uptown Girl' – before she flashed that inimitable smile and left.

Our paths crossed a few times in her glittering era, principally because the Prince's Trust had appointed me as one of its first ambassadors, called upon for such duties as master of ceremonies when one of those mammoth cheques was handed over to a recipient. Excitement bubbled at one high-security function in London because of the presence of both the Prince and Princess of Wales. On flashing my ID and being admitted, I was engaged in earnest conversation with Prince Charles about Iceland and his quiet visits to the salmon banks, when a security guard approached. Tapping my elbow, he told me my wife was waiting for me at the entrance; a puzzling message, given I could see Guðrún's face just a few feet away across the room. The uniformed staff then produced the dark-haired women to whom they had referred, who continued to insist she was my wife. She evidently was not. The mystery was never solved.

The day after Diana died in 1997 programmes on Capital slipped abruptly into solemn mood, ditching the upbeat hits for ethereal music and news updates.

Chris Tarrant's familiar grin fell as he broadcast tearful messages from listeners. 'Jackie wrote to me: "With all the love we have for Diana, she will remain alive in our hearts forever and may she, at last, be at peace".' No radio station was quite prepared for the national outpourings which ensued, and London became a strange place to be, as the pile of flowers outside Kensington Palace grew. Like all major news events, you remember where you were when you heard the news. I was in hospital, having suffered an interminable nosebleed with no obvious cause. As I lay on my bed in the small hours in discomfort from the padding up my nose to stench the flow, the 'breaking news' tickertape appeared on a silent flickering TV screen at the end of the ward.

The Flying Eye was a symbol of Capital's scale and ambition. It flew over London, zig-zagging the Thames and beaming back traffic reports into peak-time programmes. These were the times when information could not be readily piped in by computer and camera feeds, nor could listeners readily contribute as mobile phones were still rare, so this lofty vantage point was invaluable. Russ Kane and David Briggs were amongst those on board, generating frequent informed reports with a sense of urgency and useful drama from fifteen-hundred feet in the air. David was a positive, nice guy, and quick to seize opportunities. Little wonder that, after rising to deputy programme director, he was to leave to join GMTV before playing a role in developing the *Who Wants To Be A Millionaire?* TV format with Celador, drawing on his experiences as a brilliant radio producer. His Capital spell afforded him excellent first-hand experience of the talents of Chris Tarrant – and a wife, when he married Jo Sandilands.

The job I do means that the lives of fascinating individuals collide with mine at key stages in their career, amounting almost to an accidental showbiz version of the TV show *7-Up*. Meeting an upbeat Genesis in 1987 at Capital when they were just about to complete their *Invisible Touch* tour with four sell-out nights at Wembley Stadium – a feat no other act had ever achieved – came in stark contrast to their early days battering on the door of Radio Luxembourg at midnight desperate for airplay. In the Seventies I asked about their hopes and dreams; by the Eighties I was asking 'How much better can it get?' in the light of their five Top 5 singles in the US. By then, Phil Collins was fronting the band, with his vivid dress sense, energy and commercialism helping to speed the journey to success. In the interview at Capital, Phil, Tony Banks and Mike Rutherford spoke to me with mature professionalism about their work, including a fascinating reference to their collegiate working, 'Like three guys with their trousers down doing it.' They were illustrating colourfully the openness of their working style, recognising that each band member can contribute ideas to a session and try them out without fear of failure.

Artists often went to great pains to thank me for playing their music. In response, I thanked them for making it. Without their music, my career would not have existed.

Stevie Wonder is a huge talent. We had first met in 1972 at Radio Luxembourg's London offices at the time of his album *Music of My Mind*, which marked a new direction for Stevie, making use of synthesisers. I loved that work, although I gather Motown founder Berry Gordy was less enthusiastic. Stevie had become blind at six weeks old owing to being placed in an incubator containing too much oxygen, yet, in my Capital days, he arrived at a function I was attending in London calling out '95.8, where are you?' It was a trick he rehearsed well. Abdul 'Duke' Fakir from the Four Tops tells of how Stevie walked up to Gladys Knight at a session in Detroit and complimented her on the colour and style of her clothes, having taken the trouble to ask his aides acting as his eyes to scout the room before his entrance to let him know exactly who and what to expect once inside.

Chuck Berry turned up forty minutes late for my interview with him. We had arranged to meet in the foyer of a swish London hotel, as he was in town connected with the production of a documentary movie. Clare, the newsroom producer, and I showed him to the table we had commandeered and he sat down, declining a drink and obstinately failing to engage in social chit-chat. When he asked how long we needed, I explained the piece was for a half-hour documentary, to which he snapped back that we would be afforded just ten minutes. When I tried to explain politely that it would be a challenge for us to do justice to his career in such a short window, he took off his watch, placed it in front of us and declared we now had nine minutes. At the end of each answer, as I began another question, he picked up his watch for inspection. He was not in a good mood that day.

Most people in radio have someone to thank for seeing an early spark of talent and giving them an early opportunity. For me, it was my scoutmaster back home and pirate broadcaster Steve Young who pointed me in the right direction, and the early bosses at Luxembourg for having faith in me. In time, it is good to be able to help others too.

Angie Greaves worked as a management secretary at Capital, and as I walked past her office door each day to get to and from the studios I often popped in to chat. We got on well and I remarked on the rich, sunny character in her voice, eventually recruiting her treacly tones to record some 'sweeper' jingles for my show. I then suggested she record an audition, which she credits as the start of her radio career which has seen her broadcast on Magic, Choice, BBC local radio, Jazz FM, LBC and Smooth. Angie deserves her success. She is a true entrepreneur and has become a voiceover in demand around the world.

Chris Tarrant joined Capital the same year I did. His tall figure had become known for his madcap messy Saturday TV antics on *TISWAS*, but I also recognised his face from the year I was living in the East Midlands. He had been a rookie contributor to the evening news magazine programme *ATV Today*, covering odd items including, memorably, the story about the man who walked from Evesham to Worcester with four ferrets down his trousers.

A maestro on radio, naturally in command of his craft, his first weekday daytime show was aired at lunchtimes after my mid-morning show, before he graduated to the breakfast show. Chris stayed as circus-master of that key early slot for seventeen hugely-successful years, becoming unassailable owing to his audience ratings. Such was his stature, he had a demonstrable personal effect on the value of the company, a huge tribute to the gifted hiring and scheduling decisions of Jo Sandilands.

Our on-air handovers were typified by the sort of brotherly teasing that good friends get away with, but our insult humour may well have alarmed infrequent listeners. He was a hard worker, who identified the huge potential of the programme and was focused on realising it. To say he took his breakfast rivalry with Chris Evans seriously would be an understatement.

Relaxed and confident in his own skin, like many greats, he was the same off-air as he was on, and also hugely compassionate. When colleagues he had come to know were going through a bad time, for example when contracts were not being renewed, it would be Chris who offered to take them out for an uplifting drink or meal. In one memorable encounter when he extended the hand of friendship to me, I was invited to a bistro-pub for a lunch hour which lasted five. Whilst the intention was to enjoy a quiet catch up, he ended up providing impromptu fringe theatre for all the staff and customers. I am thankful for his friendship.

18

THE NETWORK CHART

Since the days of *Pick of the Pops*, listening to the BBC chart early on Sunday evenings had become a British tradition. Listeners excitedly slid their C120 cassettes in their tape machines to capture the entire programme on BBC Radio 1 as the songs which were exciting the nation were played in full, building to the drama of the latest Number One.

The BBC Top 40 dominated Sunday evening radio listening. It was a big, clean machine, supported by the might of the BBC, with high-profile presenters over the years such as Alan Freeman and Tony Blackburn, and by TV's *Top of the Pops*.

Commercial radio attracted comparatively small audiences that time of the weekend, but there was an ambition that a new generation of national chart show could harvest greater listener enthusiasm. The then-regulator, the Independent Broadcasting Authority, was more cautious, declaring in 1979 that it believed a 'networked pop programme… goes against the spirit of ILR (Independent Local Radio).'[18]

Most stations at the time were owned by proud independent local companies and shared little programming, in stark contrast to the consolidated commercial radio industry we recognise today.

The Network Chart eventually launched on Sunday, 30th September 1984, shortly after my move to Capital, with the vision

---

18 IBA statement January 1979; *Crossing the Ether*, Sean Street.

of creating a programme aired across the entire commercial radio network. At the outset it was carried by the vast proportion of stations – forty-four of the forty-eight, 'From Edinburgh's Radio Forth to Bristol's Radio West – you know it makes sense, this chart is the best.' Aside from the questionable poetry, the first edition compared rundown positions with the trial programme from the preceding week, with Elton, Bucks Fizz and, as I regretfully said, 'Heaven One-Seven' falling out the chart.

The show relied on a chart compiled by MRIB (Media Research & Information Bureau), calculating its positions by taking radio station airplay into account alongside record sales. This was sound thinking, already adopted in the US by the Billboard chart, but not the BBC/Gallup chart which still drew on sales figures alone at the time, just as the first-ever record chart had done in 1952 when *NME* founder Percy Dickens phoned twenty record shops to see which discs were faring well. Record buyers and radio listeners, however, are not the same people. A record could be momentarily popular with young record buyers and rise high up the charts, yet not be particularly well-received by listeners at large. The Number One song on both UK charts was, however, usually the same.

As I prepared to go on-air one week, my producer Tony Hale affixed a sign to the studio wall in front of me which read 'Why should anyone listen to me?', and quizzed me for a decent answer. That powerful sign was stuck up every week afterwards – a reminder that radio is not about the presenter, it is about the listener.

Aside from the different data it leaned on, the winning formula for the show was its pace and tone, inspired by the energy of Sky Sports TV presentation. I was flattered to learn later of the irony that the team at Sky Sports were using tapes of my chart to coach their new presenters. To me, the battle of the bands to reach the top spot, their rival audiences cheering them on, the tension of the wait for the whistle to blow at Number One – and the moment of victory and parallel disappointment – all mirrored the speed and emotion of sport. It is probably also why the programme trailers for sports programmes on TV and radio now routinely hijack the emotion of music to accompany the clips. I was asked whether I might try sports commentary myself, feeding my interest in the field, but my manager at the time suggested it was not the right career move. Whilst he likely had his reasons, I know not what they were.

Addressing a national audience on their local stations carries some risk. Birmingham is not Manchester; Edinburgh is not Portsmouth. Tony quite liked me calling the show 'the Netty', as it sounded pithy and affectionate and may have caught on with the audience. Not in Newcastle, though, where we were told it means a toilet. In a similar vein, announcing new entries in the chart as coming 'in with a bullet', one of those familiar phrases from the chart show lexicon, went down poorly in a still troubled Belfast. After a polite intervention from Downtown Radio, I never said it again. Constructive feedback generally was always welcome, but trying to please all the different programme directors across all the stations was akin to a bucking bronco ride.

The Network Chart was the underdog, and tried harder because of that. The show amassed support from the record labels, who valued a competitor for the BBC, and they seemed to appreciate its fresher, energetic approach. This was a time when the BBC as a whole was victim of one of the periodic onslaughts, with speculation even extending to the suggestion that Radio 1 should be privatised, prompting the *Sun* to report that 'David Jensen's Chart Show on the commercial radio network is slicker and more up to date then the BBC equivalent.'

Alongside the hits, the programme was spiced with artists' voices and pre-produced audio drop-ins, in contrast to the BBC's more functional format at the time. The stars themselves seemed to enjoy the programme, and it was great to learn from the head of Columbia promotions that he had been asked by Daryl Hall, lead vocalist from Hall and Oates, to post off a copy on cassette each week. At a time when we were very much the newcomer, I was always flattered, if a little surprised, when opinion-formers suggested they were choosing our offering over the established alternate.

The chart attracted fans in the radio industry. One night, having finished dinner at Kenny Everett's house, he stood up and asked, 'What do you think of this?', in the way only Kenny could, before flinging open a filing cabinet drawer to reveal meticulously-labelled tapes of every edition of my programme.

As far as critical acclaim is concerned, Clive James, whom I admired, did pen one review which was a little lukewarm, with the sting in its tail '…right down to its Canadian host.' I had clearly been the last straw. On arrival in the UK, I had often been asked generally if I felt my accent would be an asset, or a millstone around my neck. Thankfully, I feel it has proven usefully distinctive, and I was reassured at the outset by the national treasure status afforded to the Australian Alan Freeman, the guardian of the BBC's *Pick of the Pops* programme. Perversely, on my occasional visits to Canada my accent is now discerned to be British.

In its early days, our show relied on a wire rack of thirty vinyl discs, and was broadcast live. Countdown programmes sound simple on-air, but the necessary precision means they are demanding to deliver, as every chart show host will attest. The pace and drama must be built in very few words, and the sort of adlibbed asides that get you out of trouble in routine conversational programmes stand out as they might were the Queen to go off-piste in her Christmas message. The other key challenge is nailing complex timing, not least in pre-digital days where calculations were engineered only with the aid of a stopwatch and hasty maths. The right amount of time must be allotted to play all the relevant songs in their entirety in the right order. I might be forgiven, therefore, for the one occasion when I played the Number One at the wrong speed – an error which has now thankfully reached virtual obsolescence.

In latter days, *The Network Chart* was pre-recorded and used CDs, before moving to digital music playout. Despite being broadcast on both FM and AM, the programme used low-quality landlines to convey the programme to each city's station in the days before satellites, and thus it was heard by listeners only in struggling mono. By contrast, BBC Radio 1, which was routinely transmitted only on AM in mono, borrowed Radio 2's FM frequencies for Sunday evenings, so its Top 40 could be enjoyed in juicy stereo. Richard Skinner took the helm of the BBC's offering from Simon Bates on the day my chart was launched; and, despite the inferior audio quality of our offering, we spared no effort in competing with this grand institution.

Besides the hard work on-air, promotional effort was important and Capital's Flying Eye Traffic Plane was hijacked so I could journey around the country to visit local host stations. The simplicity of its navigation concerned me. When I asked the pilot where we were, he just pointed down to the M1 winding below us.

As well as meeting listeners, the travels around the country helped all the partners in the network feel part of the venture and embrace the show more enthusiastically on-air. Some proud local stations were only reluctantly donating two hours of their treasured local Sunday programming time in favour of this content 'from London', but any management suspicion appeared to be readily assuaged by the prospect of a stream of new revenues. We also bribed our hosts with generous boxes of assorted orange and white sweatshirts, T-shirts and mugs – the sort of lavish merchandising which many could not afford at the time for their own stations.

On one of these trips I met Paul McKenna, in his days at Chiltern Radio. Paul has carved out a gigantic worldwide career as a hypnotherapist, but back then he was a radio presenter in Dunstable with a great voice and huge ambition. Always chatty and entertaining, he had a fund of stories which he delivered brilliantly. I gather others quickly identified the worldwide success he would achieve, but at the time I just took him as he was – a good guy. As his second career began to take off, I recorded a bunch of announcements for him to introduce his stage act, playing to his love of the Atlantic style of radio.

He was a practical joker too, and took delight in phoning up during songs whilst I was on-air to challenge me to incorporate a rude word discreetly in the next link; utterly childish fun we both thoroughly enjoyed.

TV afforded a further opportunity to market the programme to fresh audiences. Erasure performing 'Victim of Love' kicked off *The Roxy*, a series I hosted in 1987 produced by Tyne Tees TV. Subtitled *The Network Chart Show*, it was based on the same chart as the radio show. An array of comedians co-hosted, with appearances from Ben Elton, Rik Mayall and Adrian Edmondson, an innovative idea at a time when comedians were not generally seen as hosts and entertainers in the way they are now.

One risk of being in the public eye is the annoyance of picking up a newspaper and reading reports stating you have said or done something you have not. A producer of *The Roxy* had fed a line to a press reporter suggesting I had said the show would 'blow *Top of the Pops* out the water.' A journalist put my alleged comment to Mike Hurll, the *Top of the Pops* producer, who responded with atypical but understandable brusqueness. I regret I never seized an opportunity to reassure him it was not what I believed, and make clear the high regard I still had for the team and for him. Michael died in 2012.

The Roxy, however, was to end with a whimper – it had not started with much of a bang either. Artists sometimes were reluctant to travel up to Tyne Tees to appear; there was an industrial dispute, and the programme was shunted around the schedule inhibiting any growth in audience loyalty. When some of the then separate ITV companies chose to stop carrying it at all, it died after just nine months.

The radio show continued to thrive. In its first six months on-air it had virtually doubled the Sunday afternoon audience for the network, and I was delighted to win the title 'UK Radio Personality of the Year'[19] in the 1985 Sony Radio Awards.

Besides growing audiences, the *Network Chart Show* lent commercial benefits to what was still a young and fragmented industry. Booking radio advertising campaigns across the whole country was then a complex affair as each station was independent – and its format and audience different. Sophisticated advertisers were not wholly tempted by that piecemeal offering, hence national revenues for the industry overall were not being optimised. *The Network Chart* offered a simple coherent programme environment which advertisers easily understood and in which they could buy ad spots with ease.

In the early days, De Beers diamonds were a major spender. At that stage, although the demanding rules meant the company was not allowed strictly to sponsor the programme, the client booked campaigns throughout each show giving the impression it belonged to them. The strategy made sense, and they successfully marketed diamonds for all purposes from graduation to engagement and weddings.

Capital often called upon the halo of its presenters to help seal major commercial deals. A few months after launch I was wheeled out to entertain the boss of Nescafé over a fine dinner. Although I never felt I could master the science of selling, I did feel the on-air

19 IBA Yearbook,1986.

team had a part to play in lubricating the process. We chatted over the show and thankfully got on well. As with so much in sales it is about relationships, so it was good that we could talk football – and he supported Crystal Palace. He signed the initial agreement – and subsequent ones – and the programme was badged *The Nescafé Chart Show* when the regulations eventually permitted.

When you have seen the whites of the client's eyes, you understand how much the deal means to them and, when on-air, you go the extra mile when delivering the show and the client credits. As part of the deal, I also helped Nescafé as a brand ambassador with some their activities and undertook contractually that, whenever I was seen, I always drank coffee – and always theirs. Over the course of a decade, at the behest of sponsors, my public hot beverage loyalties had to shift from the Tea Council's products whilst at Radio Luxembourg to the aroma of coffee on commercial radio.

Nescafé remained committed, sponsoring the programme for eight years until 1993.

After I ceased presenting it, the Chart Show, in its various incarnations, continued to grow in stature over the years and, like a proud parent whose children flee the nest, I cheered its later victories. By 2015 commercial radio reached over two million listeners at 6.00 on a Sunday night, compared with half a million for Radio 1, which then shunted its rundown to midweek. Although the charts on commercial radio have now gone their separate ways, with the major groups ploughing their own furrow on Sunday evenings, it was great to have built the foundations of a programme which played such a key role in the industry's fortunes for well over thirty years.

19

BATTLE OF THE BANDS: THE BEATLES

As I wandered through Kenny Everett's Gold studio one day, as I routinely did on the way to my Capital FM chair, he turned the volume down on the speakers to greet me and our chitchat turned to holidays. 'Peter Island in the British Virgin Islands,' he hissed. 'That's where you need to go. You've earned enough money from all those gigs.'

Just a few weeks later, having taken Kenny's recommendation, my family and I were happily enjoying a fortnight away, relishing the peace of that heavenly Caribbean island.

One morning, as we walked in the sun along the perfect white sand, I heard a voice cry out 'It's the Kid!'

The voice belonged to Paul McCartney. Whenever he saw me, he always pointed at me with two fingers in a pretend gun motion and uttered those Wild West words with a theatrical furrowed brow.

There were very few villas on the island but, coincidentally, he was occupying one too – equipped, naturally, with a piano which had been lifted in by crane from a boat and installed just for his purposes.

Our sunny encounter was wholly unexpected, but our families got on well and we found ourselves back at his villa, just sharing McCartney family life with a relaxed and jokey Paul. His then wife Linda was an angel, with the knack of making sure a room full of strangers all became friends by the end of the night. We spent a good deal of time together over the break, and I picture us sitting on his daughter Stella's single bed listening to tracks from his new album *Press to Play*, which bore the romantic sepia picture of him and Linda on the cover. At random moments like that, it's easy to be starstruck. Imposter syndrome kicks in, and the thought goes through your mind; 'That's Paul McCartney – why am I here?' But the biggest names do not want you to feel like that; they like to behave normally, and they want you to do the same.

Our paths collided many times over the years. In the mid-Seventies days of Wings, the McCartneys invited us to a family dinner at their home in Battle, East Sussex. Linda served up a Sunday roast lentil dish, given her credentials as an animal rights activist and vegetarian advocacy. Our children and theirs are of similar ages, so it was a chilled day of go-kart track building, going for a walk in the woods and fooling around.

Paul had bought a Speak and Spell game for Stella, which I asked about, impressed by the neat technology for the time. When I expressed surprise that this multi-millionaire knew exactly how much the toy cost from Foyles, he explained how important he felt it was to keep a sense of value, whatever your earnings.

On another occasion we attended a dinner as their guests, with our growing families spread across two adjacent tables. Just after the main course, Linda came across, hands on hips and expression stern, having just been chatting to my daughter. 'I cannot believe what I've just heard. You make Anna Lisa eat meat!' she remonstrated. 'She'll tell me if you feed her that again.' From far across the table came a Cheshire cat grin from my daughter, who had clearly been discussing the merits of vegetarianism with her new allies.

Paul supported my professional efforts, for which I was always grateful. At the Live 8 concert in Hyde Park in 2005 hosted by Bob Geldof, Paul was on the bill alongside around thirty other acts from Madonna to Coldplay, Elton and the Who, kicking off singing 'Sgt. Pepper's Lonely Hearts Club Band' with U2 and finishing performing immaculately alongside George Michael. Backstage, word got around that Paul would speak to one of the assembled journalists hungry for a headline. He duly appeared, walking through the area where the world's media waited, scanning his eyes around. Our eyes met; and off I was taken to conduct the major interview. On my return, sated, the serious journalists gathered around me in the hope I might give them the news lines they needed. That was a good feeling.

Paul appeared in a TV series I hosted called *Afternoon Club,* a chat programme launched by TVS at a time when the channel was seeking to curry favour with viewers after controversially daring to abandon its afternoon horse-racing coverage. After the programme, I bumped into him again in the car park and we chatted in the sunshine. After the usual pleasantries, he asked whether I minded some honest feedback about what I do on radio. You do not turn down advice from Paul McCartney; and his words were insightful. He suggested I would be more successful were I to talk on-air a little more about my own life and perspectives, suggesting that he learned so much more about me over the dinner table than he did from my programmes. To hijack Alan Keen's Radio Luxembourg phrase, I had always worried whether listeners really were interested in how my tomatoes were growing, but I was learning that the relationship between listener and presenter is a little different in the UK. John Peel offered much the same advice, and I tried to take it on-board, although truly being yourself on-air is a real art. I know of several broadcasters whom listeners have yet to witness how entertaining they really are.

I do not recall making a disparaging remark about the work of the Beatles whilst on-air at Capital. It had been reported to Paul, however, that I had. It was simply a misunderstanding, but he called off an interview the next day, and our relationship cooled for a year or two. Thankfully, our paths then crossed during a function held at the BFI in Piccadilly. As I walked in, he was standing at the top of the stairs with his second wife, Heather Mills. Paul's hand came out his pocket with the familiar two finger gun gesture, and he gave the familiar 'It's the Kid' cry. We had made up.

I respect him hugely.

Ringo and I spoke a few times at the height of his career, and I found him a thoroughly down-to-earth guy, just living the dream. When the Beatles were promoting *Abbey Road* at the end of 1969, I was offered the chance of an interview with him at Apple records. I picture myself waiting in the dark reception area of the Savile Row building which, earlier that year, had seen the famous rooftop concert which was their final live performance. Mary Hopkin walked through and climbed the stairs, followed later by Paul McCartney. Eventually, Ringo popped down, wearing a floppy velvet hat. 'David! Come upstairs,' he said. 'Excuse my hair, it needs washing – it's greasy.' It is the small things that stick in your mind.

In the interview, aired on Radio Luxembourg on the September day *Abbey Road* was released, Ringo took me through the album track by track. He suggested they had thrown around abstract names for many weeks before Paul suggested *Abbey Road*, recognising simply where the EMI studios, which had spawned the recording sessions, were sited. None of the Beatles had a better idea, so it stuck. Ringo also spoke casually of the album cover: 'We stood in Abbey Road and had our photo taken for it. EMI's just ahead of the Volkswagen, folks.' Little did he know when we were speaking that Iain Macmillan's photograph would become iconic. The zebra crossing would be awarded Grade II listed status, and EMI studios would be re-named Abbey Road Studios.

He heaped praise on George Harrison for 'Something': 'Best track on the album.' As I put the needle on the vinyl and aired it on 208 that night over fifty years ago, it was the first time most people across Europe ever heard the Ivor Novello award-winning melody which is now part of our musical heritage.

I believe George Harrison was never given due credit for his trailblazing work on guitar, using amplification and sound effects long before anyone else. He was a lovely, friendly, gentle guy who loved his music. He also shared my passion for motor racing, and our paths had crossed when we were both guests of the Williams team. I confess when he was a guest on my show and we played a Beatles song, I used to turn it down on the studio speakers so we could just chat amongst ourselves about who would win the Grand Prix.

Alas, John Lennon was a missed opportunity. As a young presenter at Radio Luxembourg, I had been given the chance of a real exclusive: chatting to him down-the-line in New York at the time he was battling with US authorities and risked deportation owing to his conviction following his 1968 drugs raid. It was a Sunday night, and the recording had been scheduled just before my bingo show. This was a huge moment, and it was no surprise that my colleague Tony Prince asked if he could listen-in as we chatted.

The combination of Lennon on the phone and being watched by a more experienced presenter gave me an attack of the nerves I had never had before and have never suffered since. Here was one of the biggest interviews of my career, and I just could not face it. Tony volunteered to take over.

Listening in the adjacent studio as the call came through, I heard John's familiar Liverpool accent: 'Hi, is that Kid?'

I kicked myself.

20

BATTLE OF THE BANDS: THE BEACH BOYS

'Brian Wilson's waiting for you downstairs,' said my Capital producer, having just taken a puzzling call from the station's reception. As I was not expecting the co-founder of the Beach Boys to appear on my programme that day, or indeed to wander into reception, I dismissed the message repeatedly as a joke.

But the heavy blue studio door opened, and the real Brian walked in. Friendly, but staggering a little and looking a touch dishevelled, he was accompanied by a guy with long blond hair who looked a little like one of WWE wrestlers. He was Eugene Landy, the American 'shrink to the stars', known for his unconventional ways. Brian introduced him as his doctor and asked if he could sit in for our impromptu interview.

We talked about his recently-released new solo album, *Love and Mercy*, but I equally wanted to explore his relationship with, and treatment from, the guru by his side who'd taken control of his life, monitoring him around the clock and treating him to fend off the drugs and junk food.

Maybe scarred from the experience of my over-eager questions suffocating the Van Morrison interview, I afforded Brian all the time he needed for this Capital conversation. I thought that if he needed ten seconds before answering a question then the listeners should hear that pause for thought.

Brian is often thought of as the lead voice on the searing harmonies of 'God Only Knows' from *Pet Sounds*, but that belonged to his younger brother Carl. Brian once said to me: 'You know who's the proper singer in this band, the real singer? The one with the best voice? Carl.'

I first met Carl when he came over to Radio Luxembourg, promoting his solo album *Carl and the Passions: So Tough*. I also saw him socially once or twice in London and in Los Angeles, and we genuinely enjoyed each other's company. Bearded, he looked a little like a disciple of the Maharishi, a truly sweet-natured, ordinary guy with a special gift.

Carl invited me over for dinner at his home, a contemporary and stylish villa, but not flashy, which was not far from his brother's. As we paused between courses, his wife sorting the dessert, he told me he wanted me to listen to something. Adjourning to another room, he slid in a cassette and I prepared myself to be treated to some exciting new work, but Carl looked concerned.

On the first tape, we heard just the opening notes of the Kinks' 'You Really Got Me' being played repeatedly. He explained these were Brian's recordings. He put another tape in the deck, this time bearing the first notes of 'Be My Baby' from the Ronettes, again edited together addictively. Carl turned to me; 'This is what he does. What would you feel if your brother did this?' He was evidently concerned for his brother's prevailing mental state. I tried to reassure as best I could; Brian could clearly count on a brother who cared.

Famously, as depicted in the film *Love and Mercy*, it was suggested that Brian felt he would be more inspired to produce songs if he were on the beach, but did not want to go there, so he built a low wall round his dining room and filled it deep with sand onto which a grand piano was placed.

My most recent meeting with Brian saw him on better form, on stage at the Royal Festival Hall in connection with an album called *Smiley Smile*, which was my wife Guðrún's favourite Beach Boys album. The record label had arranged that we could both catch up with Brian after the show, although an officious representative dispensed a list of instructions on arrival: 'You can see Brian at the end of the show. But there is no hand touching. No conversation. No interviews. No hidden microphones. There is none of that crap.'

Given the meeting was sounding increasingly like visiting Father Christmas in Harrods, Guðrún was not impressed. As we approached, Brian got up slowly, a lumbering physical guy, and offered his hand. I could hardly refuse the gesture, despite the lengthy briefing. On the strength of that, I ventured to introduce Guðrún and he enquired where she was from. After exchanging a few cordial words about Iceland, with the PR person glowering a few feet away, Guðrún asked for a photograph. 'Sure,' said Brian, ensuring we had as many as wanted. As Guðrún walked out the room ahead of me, I followed with Brian by my side. He placed his hand on my shoulder and said under his breath, 'She's good vibes, man. Good vibes.'

21

LIVE AID

You remember where you were the day of Live Aid.

It was a sticky hot July day in 1985. Bob Geldof and Midge Ure spearheaded the world's biggest benefit event for the Ethiopian famine, a cause which had touched them as it touched so many of us. Michael Buerk's powerful BBC News report called it 'a biblical famine in the 20th century' when the anticipated rains failed for the sixth successive season, and a crisis became a catastrophe.

Who can now hear 'Drive' by the Cars without picturing that distressing footage of desperate skeletal children in rags clinging to their mothers, watching with expressionless eyes, flies landing on their faces in the baking heat?

The event was staged simultaneously at the JFK stadium in Philadelphia and Wembley Stadium in London. I was one of the seventy thousand people who attended in England, with a worldwide TV audience estimated at around 1.5 billion in sixty countries delivered by an unprecedented web of international satellites. It was to change the face of charity fundraising.

The event was a logistical triumph, with over seventy-five artists on the bill from David Bowie to Paul McCartney, Phil Collins to Ultravox, Spandau Ballet to U2. Owing to the sheer number of performers, each one largely lingered in their trailers close to the stage waiting for their allotted time rather than backstage, the accommodation being handed over once the performance was complete to make way for the next acts.

Status Quo had the privilege of kicking off the event. I was in their van beforehand with Francis Rossi, Rick Parfitt and Alan Lancaster. It was Pete Kircher's final performance with the band. The mood was one of chatting and joking; the sort of garrulousness which is often a cover for anxiousness.

Richard Skinner from Radio 1 began the proceedings. 'It's twelve noon in London, seven am in Philadelphia, and around the world it's time for Live Aid.'

After the Coldstream Guards played the National Anthem, Quo took to the stage. I had expected to introduce them, but the plan changed – and Griff Rhys Jones and Mel Smith, dressed as police officers, brought the guys on. Now a Capital presenter rather than a BBC figure, I suspect I was less likely to be chosen for such duties.

As Quo struck up 'Rockin' All Over The World' the day was underway, the largest music event ever in the world. The picture of a moustached and muscular Freddie Mercury in his white vest became the iconic picture of the day, as he kicked off Queen's twenty-one minutes of superlative performance. All the acts raised their game – even the audience were not just watching, they were part of it.

The youngest performer on the London stage across the whole day was Steve White, drummer with the Style Council. It was great to see how well he had done, with his relationship with the band having begun when he was invited to play with them on a session for my Radio 1 show.

All taking part were militarily organised, as was necessary to ensure that each performer got on stage at the right time, for the right amount of time, with all the right sound equipment. This would be a shining light on any artist's CV, and it was important to get it right for a host of reasons. For U2, it was the performance which truly broke them.

Aside from the magnitude and significance of the event, the venue itself added to the electricity of the occasion. For those into both their music and their football, performing on the turf where England won the World Cup in 1966 was a special moment. I spoke to Brian May a few months later for *The Way It Is* on Capital, and he commented the venue did 'move your bowels a bit' that day.

It was reported that Live Aid raised forty million pounds for Africa, with half of the money spent on food and half on long-term development.

22

TROUBLESOME TV

Kenneth Williams certainly made an impression. As we waited in the wings for a TV appearance, he looked at me accusingly. 'You're American, aren't you?' he asked with disdain and a Williams nose-wrinkle. 'Canadian,' I replied, in my defence. 'Doesn't matter. Same thing,' he huffily retorted, before moving towards me and whispering in my ear: 'Everyone here knows I've got a huge knob.' And off he walked.

Whilst radio brought its share of surprises, television brought me into contact with a whole new coterie of performers and fascinating formats.

'Don't do it,' my trusted friends advised, when I mentioned I was entertaining an offer to host a late-night series made by TVS for Anglia called *Relationships*. The concept, put to me during my time at Capital, was that we would speak openly to an adult audience about all manner of intimate topics. What could possibly go wrong?

Psychotherapist, broadcaster and author Phillip Hodson was appointed as the expert dispensing advice, and the programme was co-hosted by several women across the series, including the journalist Mariella Frostrup, TV-am presenter Jayne Irving, columnist and film critic Samantha Norman, and Sophie Aldred, who'd portrayed Dr Who's seventh companion, Ace.

On one show, around Valentine's night, we planned to turn the tables and planned a romantic surprise for my co-host of the time. Being made aware that her gentleman friend was about to propose to her, we felt it would be a lovely crescendo for the show to stage the engagement moment live on-air. Her chap showed us the ring he had bought, and the crew grew excited about what was to follow. As we brought him on to the set, however, her face fell, and when I began to explain to viewers what was about to happen, she shuffled uncomfortably. 'Will you marry me?' he asked. 'Not likely,' she said, walking off set and throwing down the ring. All I could do is bring on Phillip to discuss unrequited love.

Maybe my TV work has been more trouble-prone than radio. There was another programme about those people who go to supermarkets not to top up their shopping, although they do carry around a wire basket as an alibi, but to find love – or prepare to make love. One interviewee I talked to over the frozen peas proudly declared that she had 'taken lots of men up the aisle.'

Another show I hosted was devised by a production company headed by Michael Rodd, former presenter of *Tomorrow's World*, the popular long-running TV series on new developments in science and technology. He brought me in to chair a programme on drugs in which celebrities told the stories of their dependence and how they addressed it, generously taking viewer calls off-air after their appearance.

I glanced down at my running order on what was becoming a fast-changing, fast-moving live programme. 'John Hurt', it said. There was little time to request useful detail, before the BAFTA award-winning actor was hurried onto the set and I shook his hand quickly just before the commercial break ended. 'You are one of my favourite actors,' I told him truthfully, having seen him in such films as *Midnight Express, The Elephant Man* and the *Naked Civil Servant*. 'Thank you,' he replied, smiling. 'You're doing a great job tonight, and if I can help in any way, I'm happy to.' I assured him that we simply wanted honesty about his own situation, so viewers could relate to it and learn from his journey.

He looked aghast. 'I've not got a drugs problem and never have had,' he said icily – and truthfully. 'Counting down. Five, four, three...' the director's cue in my earpiece told me there was little time for a change of plan, and we were about to go live.

I welcomed John on-air and tried to shift the conversation immediately to safer allied territory. 'You must have met a number of people in your career who have struggled with...' 'No,' he replied. I tried again. 'In Hollywood, I imagine you probably met several colourful characters who would wrestle with...' 'Not in my experience,' he answered, stony-faced. Thankfully, he was more than eager to plug his new movie, which we quickly did.

The Miss World contests were a simpler affair, as my job was away from the camera simply being the 'voice of God', bellowing a fitting introduction to the various elements of the proceedings from my vantage point some way from the stage. I was invited by the Morleys to play my part in the huge events in major stadia in Poland, South Africa and, on two occasions, China. The event coverage in that era was mounted by a British production company, hence my involvement.

The contest has always been subject to controversy for a range of reasons, and I was nearly another part of it whilst in China. During my first week there, whilst exploring with Guðrún I innocently tried to take a tourist photograph which happened to have a submarine in shot – and another of some people being taken off a ship in handcuffs. On both occasions, my camera was confiscated by fearsome wiry military guys.

Music awards ceremonies on TV used to be more modest affairs than those of today. The British Rock and Pop Awards, the precursor to the glitz of the Brits, were originally a spin-off from the comfortable early evening BBC *Nationwide* magazine programme. I hosted the awards in 1978 with regional TV presenter Bob Wellings, in 1983 with 'newcomer to Nationwide' Anne Diamond, and in 1984 on BBC1 with Sarah Kennedy at

London's Lyceum ballroom.

Boy George carried off the *Daily Mirror* Readers' Award for 'Outstanding music personality' at the 1983 ceremony. At the height of his popularity in a year where his mantlepiece was overflowing with accolades, he earned a huge round of applause as he slowly climbed to the stage in a fetching red outfit and glittering long earrings. It was great to have him there in person, as he always has something entertaining to say when the mood is right.

Alas, I barely had time for a single question for this deserved victor in a key category before I was instructed by the director to move on. Naturally, however, it is the person in front of the camera who gets the blame for being curt. When George returned to the stage later for the duty of handing over an award to a fellow artist, I tried to make amends by congratulating him once more, but wise now to the risk, he took charge and grabbed the microphone from me, 'before you pull the mic away from me like last time...' At awards ceremonies, these are the moments which earn the column inches in the following day.

Alongside an array of TV shows from the late-night topical discussion programme *Central Weekend* to *Get Fresh* for ITV, one of the most unusual I presented was *Lumberjacks OK!*, a series of programmes about the lifestyle and history of Canadian lumberjacks produced for Channel 4. The series featured a famous contest where the guys take on all-comers in a sort of gruelling *It's a Knockout* for lumberjacks. Although I had lived in Canada, my home was some way from the deep forest, hours from civilisation where these guys spend their whole lives. The top lumberjacks earn a fortune – but have little to spend it on.

My heart will always remain in radio, but I did derive some pleasure from reading that at one stage the two most watched British TV entertainment exports were ones I was involved in: *Miss World* and *Gillette World Sports Special.*

I nearly appeared in one of the many Titanic movies, playing a role which had little to do with my radio heritage. One Saturday morning, I duly turned up for audition at a busy large rehearsal room in Soho. Surrounded by many known names, I was hustled away to show my skills in front of a small panel who briefed me on the minor part. I was to portray a tennis player on the voyage to his first overseas tennis tournament who suddenly noticed the perilous state of the ship. The character was aged 16; I was about 28. After being given the cue to start the improvisation, I gave a performance as wooden as the chair I sat on. The part rightly went to someone else.

23

CAPITAL MUSIC POWER

It was Kenny Everett who introduced me to the Filofax, the diary which was to become a symbol of Yuppie '80s life. As a record played, he called me up during my Capital Radio programme, teasing 'You'll never guess what I've got!' He just loved to be first with anything new, with a predictable penchant for electronic gadgetry. How sad to recognise that we lost him over a decade before he was able to play with even the first iPhone.

Kenny had returned to Capital from the BBC just before I joined, having also been at Euston Tower in the early days, hosting the breakfast show and then weekend programmes. He was two people rolled into one, and little like the buffoons he portrayed on TV. Calm, shy and very generous, he was also supremely entertaining. No dinner party was as good as one where Kenny turned up. He regaled us with stories until we were convulsed with laughter, and his chemistry with his soulmate Paul Burnett was irresistible.

Kenny's latest radio home was on the new Capital Gold, which launched when Capital separated the programming on its AM and FM frequencies, which had hitherto carried the same output. He was presenting at that oldies station when the announcement came of his AIDS diagnosis, and he dealt with it typically. As I entered the studio shortly afterwards, he lay back rigid on the grey studio chair with his arms crossed on his chest, clutching a flower. 'Just practising,' he said.

I miss him. AIDS-related conditions claimed too many people

I knew in that generation. Freddie Mercury was taken aged just 45, and Andy Fraser, the bass player from the band Free who had co-written 'All Right Now' died at 62. I recall seeing Andy not long before his death, his voice wispy, his face grey and looking beyond tired. It is so sad that the gifts these talented people still had to offer will never be heard.

Aside from Kenny, Capital Gold boasted an impressive line-up of huge radio names who rode the format with skill and experience, from the indefatigable Tony Blackburn to the timeless David Hamilton, each voice as familiar to their audiences as the songs they were playing. At launch, the station had something of the air of a Sixties pirate station, promising music from 'the all-time greats' with high energy, gleeful presentation, upbeat jingles and an avalanche of Dusty, Beatles and ABBA.

The creation of the AM offshoot also allowed Capital to reinvigorate its FM service to target a complementary younger audience. In common with many of the new FM-only stations across the country, Capital FM wobbled for some time as it took off its stabilisers, with some programmes dabbling with exploratory new music before alighting on a more focussed and consistent contemporary hits-based policy. The shifts were representative of how UK radio was starting to resemble the focus of US radio, with tighter formats targeted at defined audiences.

Once it had found itself, Capital FM developed a recognisable attitude on-air. It reminded me of some of the great US radio stations, which I could hear back then only by means of cassettes posted to me from across the world in Jiffy bags. Aside from playing the great American hits of the time, the DJs over there rocked the (mixing) desk with real energy, slickness, great production values and quick humour. Like many presenters here I listened to the recordings, shaking my head in disbelief thinking that those American voices could not possibly sound that good on-air every single day. Their energy, however, inspired my own programmes, not least on those days that every presenter has where your performance does not quite sparkle the way it usually does. In the US, I concluded that the greatest DJs surfaced in the greatest radio markets. I used to think that those on air in Hawaii must be the best they could possibly get, because no-one would not want to work there.

Provocative US radio personality Howard Stern was impressed when he visited us in London, his eyebrows raising on learning the significant share of listening Capital commanded. With the benefit of both an AM and an FM service, it commanded 28% of all listening in the late Eighties, an enviable dominance by American standards. He was also taken by the studio décor, noting that 'in American radio, you can be the Number One station and still be working out of a shack.' Predictably, the recording of our chat in the studio took longer than planned and the person who had booked it next craned their neck through the door, with the familiar 'How long are you going to be?' expression on their face. 'Won't be long,' said the curly-haired legend. 'We're just two old radio guys chatting.' Being fleetingly regarded in the same peer group as one of the highest-profile and highest-earning radio personalities in the world was quite a moment.

In the Britpop days of the late Nineties, the Blur-Oasis battle was headline news and a changing political mood was felt as Tony Blair arrived in Downing Street. 'The Conservatives have been demolished,' reported BBC Radio 4 news, and the new young jeans-wearing Prime Minister seemed to fit with the national spirit of Cool Britannia.

The first ever 'battle-bus' had delivered the smiling Labour leader around the country on a whistle-stop tour as he fought that 1997 General Election campaign against John Major. It had been arranged that as the bus pulled up on the South Bank in London I would meet him to record a radio interview for Capital, and a ten-minute window had been reserved.

Tony introduced me enthusiastically to his wife Cherie. He asked how long I had been on-air, and remarked that I already seemed to have been presenting on radio 'forever'. It may have been his own enthusiasm for music dating back to his days as a wannabe rock star, and singing and playing with his band Ugly Rumours at Oxford University, but I was flattered that he seemed to know of me – even if he did not go on to say what he actually thought of my programmes.

Our paths crossed subsequently at a press awards ceremony, where again I was brandishing a mic hoping to catch something for broadcast. When he politely insisted he could not spare the time, I used the journalist's trick of asking if I might pose just a single question, resorting to a simple 'What's your favourite track of all time?' Tony paused, before smiling and replying with the name of the band he had sneaked out of Fettes school to go to see perform at the Odeon in Edinburgh in 1970. 'Deep Purple and 'Black Night'. With typical PR acumen, he then clearly questioned himself on how his choice might be greeted by the press and voters. 'Not quite sure I should be going public with that right now,' he added. It was too late.

The Capital empire was changing in a fast-moving and more competitive radio world. Famously, it was to shed several big-name presenters abruptly in a 'Night of the long knives'. Cabs were laid on outside to ferry away those whose services were no longer required once the news had been broken. Paul Burnett tells of the presenters' meeting he attended where copies of the new programme schedule were handed out, with his name absent from the daily listings. There are kinder ways to move a presenter on.

Premises lend a company some of its culture too. In 1997, Capital moved from its Euston Tower birthplace to its prestigious showbiz location in Leicester Square, a corner of town known for its red-carpet cinema premieres. A Capital-branded restaurant was even planned on the ground floor, although that venture was to be short-lived. The new premises brought clear benefits, but to me they never had the excitement and charm of Euston Tower.

Many people working in radio will suggest they are not in the business for the money. They are being truthful. Although cash can make life sweeter, most of us were simply driven at the outset of our careers – and beyond – by a hunger for a role in something special. We also want to be happy and feel valued; and, in my case, those emotions were becoming rarer at Capital.

For a small number of gifted or extremely lucky presenters, the rewards can become significant, at least for a short while, if their profiles are high and competing stations vie for their services. Most presenters on-air across the UK live peripatetic, uncertain lives earning more modest amounts – less than might be perceived. Many are also freelancers, so the security in those jobs remains only for the period of their current contract, without any redundancy benefits when they are no longer required.

At Capital, whilst I was decently rewarded, I was aware that others were earning significantly more than I was. My agent, accordingly, went into battle for a fairer settlement. His request reaped an extra three pounds a week.

24

AT LONDON'S HEART

Capital had ruled London for a generation. As the first commercial music radio station in the country, it had been allowed to stand proud and alone in one of the greatest cities in the world. The Eighties brought new commercial competitors, and the Nineties saw those blossom.

Heart 106.2 had opened in 1995, a bright red upstart with aspirations to command a significant slice of London listening. A former colleague, Keith Pringle, headed the station's programming, an animated and talented character in whom I had great faith, having known him from his days at Capital as a technical operator. I knew Kevin Palmer too, who was responsible for the music played by the fledgling station.

It was suggested that were I to transfer from Capital drivetime to host the equivalent show on Heart, my audience might hopefully follow me across. The opportunity pushed the right buttons for me, and I planned a move.

Heart in London was the second Heart station in the UK, following a year after the launch of its West Midlands sister. The stations were owned by a diversified Chrysalis, which had started life as a record company in the Sixties, founded by Chris Wright on the success of Jethro Tull's first album. I knew Chris from his connections, as an investor, in Wasps and Queens Park Rangers. He remained the chairman of Chrysalis.

The radio station was based in characterful premises out of town in West London, just on the edge of Notting Hill. At the time, the reputation for the area was not always good, as illustrated on my first ever visit when I left the building in search of some chocolate. Ahead of me, a lanky guy strutted down the road near Latimer Road Tube station. He looked around and recognised me, calling out 'It's Kid!' I shook his hand and he put his arm around my shoulder, telling me that he 'ran this area', and that I should let him know if there was anything I was concerned about. 'Free of charge, brother,' he assured me, as he walked off.

Heart was clearly a pretender to the London listening crown, although I have rarely been troubled by competitive agony. I have always simply been driven by delivering what I consider to be 'good radio'. With more stations on-air, however, the industry was naturally moving to a more adversarial position and publication of the regular audience figures, once seemingly just a matter for management closeted in offices in my early days across at Capital, had turned into a public ritual of whoops of joy, or worried faces and firings.

In 1970, whilst at Luxembourg, I was quoted by *Deejay* magazine as saying: 'Remember that in Canada or the USA a programme director will take all the DJs into a room and look at the ratings, and if you don't have top rating and you're doing the six-to-nine show they want to know why, and you leave the station if you're not doing it right. I love that.' By the time I got to Heart, that clinical approach had begun to arrive in the UK.

Showbiz was part of the DNA of the Heart brand and many figures of international renown called by, some easier to interview than others. Jennifer Lopez would have been a fine candidate had she not been surrounded by an army of minders, both accompanying her in my studio and peering through the glass from the control room. I was miffed by the needless scale of the intrusive entourage, although J.Lo seemed to do her best to have a decent conversation with me in an extraordinary environment hardly conducive to human dialogue.

At this point, in 1999, the press had been awash with tales of a fracas in a New York club involving J.Lo's then partner Puff Daddy, so I dared to ask her about the events of that night in a way which allowed her the freedom to choose how she answered. I could tell by her eyes that she was neither alarmed nor annoyed by the line of questioning, and she handled it deftly. Nevertheless, the mood in the studio grew even colder and out the corner of my eye I could see hostile exchanges in the control room between my producer and the remainder of her team. Afterwards, I was accused by her acolytes of ignoring specific instructions about the permitted lines of questioning and of 'playing the big man'. At no stage had anyone given me any such instructions.

Often, I find it is the machinery around an artist which is to blame, not the individual. On the day of Mary J. Blige's appearance she was surrounded by around ten mean-looking guys, arms folded and giving me the evil eye, almost daring me say something out of place. Mary was fine and we chatted as freely as we could, despite the menacing shadow, before the whole crew made their exit in silence without a word of farewell.

When Mary and I met again around a year later, she was accompanied just by a single helpful record company representative and the difference was palpable. She was relaxed, offering great answers to my questions. At the end she came over to whisper in my ear: 'I love to be interviewed by you.' That is how I prefer to think of her.

My goal was for interviews to be natural, genuine conversations, with any 'DJ act' turned down. I even worried about the impact of clutching a clipboard of questions, as pages of text can distract from truly listening to the answers, and even give the interviewee the impression that someone else has determined the questioning. I preferred to fly without a safety net, although it has been pointed out to me that my lifetime was my research, and I was thus instinctively familiar with much relevant background and context for many likely interviewees. Hopefully, I also knew which tougher interviewees might require just a little forethought and an aide memoire. The best tribute any broadcaster can ever receive from a listener is 'I never knew that'; when someone who has been interviewed a million times says something fresh, because the question is not copied and pasted from the same tired reference articles.

I enjoyed a couple of happy years at Heart, and the culture was certainly more relaxed than the latter days at Capital. Keith looked after me, but moved on relatively quickly to pursue an ambitious new online music venture. One challenge of any business is joining because of your faith in someone, only to see them promptly resign. New managers will then legitimately put their own stamp on the operation, as his successor as programme director Jana Rangooni did.

My lasting memory of Jana is a presenters' meeting where we assembled for the latest 'half-time' pep-talk on station plans and progress. Presenters' meetings in any radio station are usually productive in getting the team together over tea and cake, and fascinating due to the friendly clash of egos and the battle for the funniest line in any exchange. On this occasion, Jana hoisted herself up on the table and looked down on us. Walking around on the table-top, she proclaimed, 'Here I am and there are you. Who feels the more comfortable? It won't be me.' She went on to explain that her behaviour was a lesson about comfort zones. She had stepped out of hers, and she wanted to hear us on-air coming out of ours. It was a decent point, but all of us, including fellow presenter Nigel Williams in his tight lime-green cycling gear, looked on, perplexed.

Away from base, Elton John was another flamboyant character worth bumping into, exemplified by one of his birthday parties I was invited to in a New York hotel which was hosted by Robin Williams. As the rain poured down on arrival, a damp queue of dripping wet celebrities made their way through the door. Only when coats and umbrellas had been deposited did I work out to whom they belonged: Rod Stewart. KD Lang. Whoopi Goldberg. And Bill Clinton. Being Elton John must be fun.

I had rated his music for many years, personally endorsing his 1971 album *Madman Across the Water* for a Radio Luxembourg award for its standout tracks 'Levon' and 'Tiny Dancer', written about the then-wife of his songwriting partner Bernie Taupin.

We first met a couple of years later in Luxembourg, when he was promoting the album *Goodbye Yellow Brick Road*. Elton was knackered as he turned up for the interview on *Jensen's Dimensions* – the forty-seventh interview on a ten-country tour. After arriving in the Grand Duchy with his manager John Reid and grabbing a quick nap at his hotel, he came across to see us, coming alive for the interview, before being coerced to go to the Blow Up Club to meet the other DJs. Plonked in the corner before they arrived, he fell asleep. Never has anyone been seen asleep so soundly when sat on a 3kW bass bin six times their size.

Golly, the resident DJ, tried his best to awaken him with Led Zeppelin's 'Whole Lotta Love' and Sweet's 'Teenage Rampage', but to no avail. Elton repositioned his head, but his arms remained folded over his sequined chest and the Rocket Man just pulled his baseball cap further down over his head. The others arrived and a burst of Slade caused a crossing of the paisley-trousered legs, almost knocking over our Riesling '71, but still no awakening. John Reid then made his way to the DJ booth, insisting that 'Crocodile Rock' be played – at which point Golly seized the opportunity to mention he was not on DJM Records' mailing list. Elton stirred and the night progressed.

I travelled back to London on the same flight to London as Elton, who sat quietly during the journey alongside John Reid. Away from the performance, Elton was a serious operator even in those early days; a man on a mission. As his career grew, he always seemed to remember my enthusiasm for his early work, including the single 'Lady Samantha', now a collectors' item on the Philips label. That support seemed to earn me a hug when we met years later at one of his Red Piano residencies at Caesar's Palace in Las Vegas.

Chrysalis increasingly smelt the whiff of true audience victory for its Heart radio station in London, and spared no effort in understanding how listeners felt about their listening choices. It was an attention to detail I had never witnessed hitherto at Radio Luxembourg, Radio 1, or indeed Capital. Consultants were brought in from around the world, and research was studied voraciously. Francis Currie became programme director, bringing a forensic eye to the battleground. At meetings, he banged down his case and lay a watch on the table, announcing exactly how long would be permitted for any discussion. I genuinely applauded that time management. Meetings always go on too long.

For the first time in my career, strategies were shared, which is refreshing; and when consultants gave their views, the presenters were in attendance. At one meeting, it was explained to us that listeners needed to recognise a station on-air in a busy radio market instantly, within just a few seconds of hearing its music or presenters.

An A4 sheet was held up to me on a clipboard, showing some of the listeners' spontaneous comments on what they had heard on our station. My name was mentioned, which was a good sign, but the evidence suggested that listeners were persisting in referring to me as 'Kid', even though I was calling myself David on-air by this stage. The action point from that discussion was the compromise that I should become David Kid Jensen.

Some of the other findings suggested that listeners associated the way I sounded with the new rock station Virgin, rather than Heart. Privately, I could see that too; indeed, I had been talking to Virgin about opportunities.

In time, Heart reached the verdict that I was the right guy – at the wrong station. The conclusion was hammered home when I received an ominous call from my agent straight after my programme one day. Puzzled that he was calling on an internal line, I was told that he was with my boss and I should go to see them, at which point I was released from the contract. Although I understood the rationale, the termination was disarming. Having always been in control of my own destiny until that point, someone else had now chosen momentarily to seize the reins of my career journey.

Being set aside is a common experience for many presenters in what is now a trend business, with radio styles, formats and personalities coming in and out of fashion dependent on the latest thinking and competitor aggression. Sometimes that thinking is solid; at other times it may not be, so you cope in various ways. There is anger – although that achieves little – or you channel your energies into new things. You also cope by thinking of your family, recognising that, although radio is passionate territory, it is also a trade and your livelihood. But I bore no real bitterness. Although I was someone who had once been a familiar face to millions on national TV and radio – and was now out of work – I never paused to think, 'How far have I fallen?' Careers in this rich industry are more of a winding road than a mountain climb, and there are many beautiful views along the way.

25

GOLD IN THE HILLS

With its music mix and general attitude, Capital Gold in London was seeking to sound like WCBS-FM, the huge oldies station throbbing with energy across New York.

Unlike that American model, though, it puzzled me why UK oldies stations tended to limit the songs they played to the same few repetitive favourites. Surely, Elton John recorded rather more than three deserving songs. Most tracks from Michael Jackson's top-selling *Thriller* album were hugely well-known, not least because they were released as singles, yet few were played on oldies stations. Across my recent career, however, I have observed that presenters raising this very point on music repetition do so to their disadvantage.

After becoming Heartless, it was a relief to hear again promptly from Andy Turner, who had been a technical operator during my spell at Capital. He had graduated to running Capital Gold, and invited me to join him at the station. As Andy was a thoroughly nice guy, and others in the Capital building whom I regarded less highly had moved on, the offer was appealing.

June 2002 saw my return to the Leicester Square premises, hosting the late show. My first outing on Capital Gold, 'Where great music lives', featured the typical fare from Diana Ross to Roy Orbison, the Ronettes and Bryan Adams – 'the groover from Vancouver', as I believe I was first to dub him. As a seasoned presenter, it can feel odd playing oldies that you distinctly remember introducing as new releases what seems like just months before.

The debut programme also featured an exclusive interview I had secured with Lennox Lewis, the 'pugilist specialist', as he called himself, regarded by many as one of the greatest heavyweight boxers of all time. Boxing has always interested me, and it was one of the very few interests I shared with my father, whose brother had been accomplished in the field. The piece was recorded in the Poconos in Pennsylvania, with its steep mountains and cloud-covered peaks where I had spent a fascinating week as Lennox's guest, ahead of his victorious Memphis fight with Mike Tyson. The cream of the boxing fraternity were in attendance, plus many from the famous Kronk Gym in Detroit who played the part of Tyson by way of practice. Given Lennox's skills and his enormous build, he knocked them out one by one and they were stretchered off. I wondered how those fighters felt waking in the morning knowing what awaited them, rather like a procession of fated gladiators entering the Colosseum. Amidst all the testosterone, nevertheless, I watched Lennox's mood change on the day his mother arrived, as if a light had been switched on.

After being squeezed initially into the late-night programme on Gold, as that was where the gap in the schedule lay, I was shifted to mid-mornings.

A valuable initiative for the station, devised by Andy Turner, was the live performance by artists at the Café de Paris, a wonderful early-20th century venue in London's Piccadilly which had been a regular haunt for the likes of Cole Porter and later used as a backdrop for films such as *The Krays* and *Absolute Beginners*. A range of fitting Capital Gold artists appeared for us, from Jools Holland to Donny Osmond. As well as raising the station's profile and fuelling top-notch on-air ticket giveaways, they offered an opportunity for we presenters to catch up with seasoned artists and tease out a few titbits of news about them, or fresh kernels of information about the tracks they'd recorded decades before. These helped enormously on-air, addressing our daily challenge of introducing the same oldies repeatedly. Unlike more contemporary music radio formats, we never had the luxury of new releases to embrace.

Presenters do not usually need to dress up for their radio shows, so when Andy asked whether I had a tie and something smart to wear handy, the answer was no. It transpired that Prime Minister Gordon Brown was on his way to visit the Capital building. I duly rushed out to a tailor's shop down the road to purchase a modest suit, slipping on the trousers with only moments to spare.

I need not have bothered. At Leicester Square the Gold studio lay at the very end of the hallway, past the displays of all the awards and station mementos, and it was suggested the PM was not expected to venture as far as our home. A line-up of staff, however, was planned in the main office overlooking Leicester Square, so that the PM could meet the team working across the whole company. As I prepared to stand in place besides Andy, duly suited and booted, I was abruptly hustled away by company staff. Gold staff, it seemed, were not thought worthy of meeting the Prime Minister, despite the size of audience the station delivered. In Richard Attenborough's time, he would not have been ashamed of a station in the Capital stable for playing dusty old songs.

As I watched from the sidelines, the Prime Minister gave a heartfelt tribute to the medium of radio. He told how he had relied on presenters' company in his childhood and teens, and how people like us had lifted his mood and been a comfort in times of stress, such as exams. Looking at Gordon's wrinkled face and looking at the bright-eyed young things along the staff line-up, I could not help thinking that, of all of us, I was probably the only one he could possibly have listened to back then.

The commercial radio industry was in a merger frenzy. In 2005 the two large foes, the Capital group and GWR, united into one significant commercial radio player: GCap. In that new ownership structure, Capital Gold subsequently turned into simply being Gold, being carried on ever more frequencies across the UK. At that stage, I transferred to the breakfast show with Erika North, who always had boundless enthusiasm and we got on well.

Whilst I enjoyed the shows on Gold, I did not feel the love for the station I had felt for others, but it was good, at least, that some station wanted to call on my services. I tried to accentuate the positive – for the most part – even if we had to seek permission for the tiniest adjustment to programme content. Such changes would have been made by a presenter instinctively on Radio 1. I have always tried to deliver the sort of radio I want to listen to. If you are successful, you do not just inherit a station's audience, you generate new listeners who come to you because you are providing something unique.

Sadly, too, my Saturday show collided with fixtures from my other passion, Crystal Palace, and the request to Capital from my agent to record the show was not greeted favourably. It was a programme I enjoyed, nevertheless, with the station commanding an impressive guest list which included Paul Weller, Jools Holland, Jeremy Irons, Smokey Robinson, Juliette Lewis, Burt Bacharach and Tony Bennett.

Amy Winehouse featured in 2004, thanks to an unexpected encounter whilst parking my car near Wembley Arena, en-route to a gig celebrating the 50th anniversary of the Strat – the Fender Stratocaster, that renowned 1950s electric guitar. Amy was on the bill, playing bass for Jamie Cullum alongside some of the guitar giants including Gary Moore, David Gilmour and Joe Walsh. She received so much acclaim for her voice that it was easy to forget her skills as a guitarist. Amy called over to me across the street: 'Hey, you're the man with the voice.' I turned around to see the 5' 2" gifted star with her dark hair loose and dangling down almost half her height, rather than combed back into her trademark beehive style. As I smiled and acknowledged her, she emulated my delivery of the station ident: 'Music Power: Capital FM'. That night's gig was eventually released in 2005 as the film *The Strat Pack: Live in Concert*.

I introduced her on-stage a few times in her all too short career, and found her very friendly, polite and happy to help, in contrast to her reputation of sometimes being an awkward hellraiser. Amy's talent had always been clear, with her expressive, soulful, lived-in vocal sound and a compelling depth to her performance. As a person, she seemed vulnerable, lonely and in need of a good hug. I found her sincere in what she said and sang, but believe she behaved in extreme ways to get noticed and remembered. That lifestyle was to be her downfall, and the friends she mixed with were not helpful. She had a huge career in front of her – but it was sadly not to be. The music industry loses too many too soon.

The culture in the Capital building was not as pleasant or creative as it had seemed in my first spell with the Capital Group, just as the atmosphere of any company inevitably changes when it grows. Richard Attenborough's affable era of chairmanship was a fond memory, despite the tough financial challenges of his era which caused him to offer up his own paintings to the Bank of Scotland as surety so that they might advance him enough cash to pay the bills of the struggling new company.

Richard Eyre's reign was now underway. Having been managing director of Capital in the Nineties, he returned as Chief Executive of the much larger conglomeration of GCap. On arrival, he observed that the building was quieter than he had expected of a lively media organisation, and he was concerned that too little laughter echoed around its offices. He made it his mission to change GCap's reputation, so that it might move a few notches up the *Sunday Times* Best Companies to Work chart.

◉

One thing that made me happy was jazz. My father's knowledge of the genre was immense, and his appearances on radio back home in Canada were appreciated by his audiences and recognised by the jazz fraternity. With age, I grew to love it more and more, so it was a delight to be welcomed on theJazz, a digital radio station operated by GCap, which came on air at the end of 2006. One benefit from the company's expansion was its growing portfolio of stations.

In my daily show on theJazz, I played the songs my father played in his basement, and it was fulfilling, at last, to be free to play what I call 'proper jazz' from the likes of Louis Armstrong and Thelonious Monk on radio. I strike a distinction between music of that calibre and that heard on stations which appear to just nod to the genre, using any stray saxophone note as an alibi for playing almost anything. The melodies of real jazz are outstanding, and wallowing in them can be challenging, yet offer a real education into the roots of American music.

Listener comments can be much more powerful than ever they imagine. When a woman came up to me on a train and said shyly, 'I just want to say I love your station,' I reflected briefly on all those I had ever spent time at, trying to predict which she would mention. 'theJazz,' she then added, 'I really love it.' She probably did not appreciate quite how much I treasured her brief and heartfelt aside. On that station, I felt I had found myself, playing music I love and music I know about.

I regret the closure of theJazz. It was a smart radio station.

●

DAB, digital radio, was bringing many fresh new formats, offering real diversity at last to a populous country which had struggled to squeeze everything with audience potential onto the FM band.

One of the first DAB-only stations had been Planet Rock, a

passion-driven radio brand, launched in 1999. Its owner for a few years in my time was the wealthy entrepreneur and rock fan Malcolm Bluemel. He tells the story that we were sitting in a car together discussing the station's likely fate, at the time it was being sold by GCap. Such was his affection for the station as a listener, he was desperately keen that it should end up in good hands. So, rather like Victor Kiam in the famous 1980s Remington shaver TV ad, he liked the company so much, he bought it. It was reported he had won the station's ownership in the face of interest from other artists, including Queen's Brian May.

Attracting over a million listeners these days, its line-up over the years has included Alice Cooper, Def Leppard's Joe Elliott, and my old Capital colleague Nicky Horne.

I enjoyed my three years on-air at Planet Rock in Malcolm's tenure. Despite the change of ownership, it still lodged in GCap's premises, with desks in the open plan offices where his enthusiasm was clear to see, and was reflected by its presenters.

On my Saturday show on the station I was joined by Rick Wakeman, a natural on radio as a compelling raconteur, and truly one of the most quick-witted guys I know. Our programme was wholly ad-lib, and I confess not a single word was prepared in advance. On the road, he had been the life and soul of the party; first at the bar, holding court with an impressive array of familiar music names… and he recounted colourful tales on-air of those days. Once the microphone was switched off, he told me the juicy bits of the stories he had chosen to miss out. It was good to see that he had sensibly calmed down a little since the heady days from which his tales sprung, as we all must.

Rick's reputation is enormous, and when on the road now with other Yes alumni in what he calls 'the Yes tribute act', the gigs are massive, selling out years in advance. Not only is he a great musician, he is a good businessman and a thoroughly caring guy; one of those characters with a filing cabinet between his ears and the enviable gift of remembering who everyone is and what they do.

Sadly, Planet Rock remained a tough financial challenge as a stand-alone brand, and Malcolm Bluemel disposed of it to Bauer Media in 2012, in whose hands it remains on-air.

My day-job at Gold edged to a close too, and I walked out the doors of the Capital empire once more. The farewell was decent this time, with champagne, snacks and reminiscences. I was to miss the support team and producers and the general environment of the station, although it had been different from places I worked at earlier in my career. Production staff had broader listening horizons, rather than just the station they worked on and, although they possibly did not have Gold running through their veins as the Luxembourg team had for their station in an unrepeatable era, there was a laudable objectivity and professionalism.

26

CHANGE IN THE AIR

When I posted a letter to Radio Luxembourg in 1968, armed just with little experience and a bundle of hope, I had no idea what the future would bring. From that moment on, the momentum of my career never stopped. For decades, someone always stepped forward to present enticing new opportunities to me. I have been truly fortunate.

Now, the ambitious Kid Jensens of today should – and will – get their time to shine; and I would not wish to stand in their way. I love doing what I do, however, and feel I have something still to offer even if, more recently, I have needed to bang on doors personally to secure the opportunities across a merry-go-round of formats.

Smooth Radio was my next stop in 2011. Back then, the station was housed in Salford, where I joined an outrageously funny team whose company I enjoyed. I stopped over there for four days each week and often bumped into familiar faces in the media hub the area was becoming. The station afforded me a surprisingly impressive pied-à-terre: a spacious corner apartment high up at Media City, from where the glittering view of the night-time sky made Manchester look like Vegas. Nicky Campbell envied me from the more modest and typical apartment in which he was accommodated.

I felt highly-regarded at Smooth, and was sometimes called upon to be questioned in front of an invited audience, making use of my catalogue of radio and music tales as a sideshow at events organised to help clients feel favourably about the station. I hope my veteran appearances helped make a useful contribution, but, in honesty, it was simply good to feel valued, in sharp focus to the way I felt presenters were viewed and treated elsewhere.

Today's presenters are commercially-savvy and, at last, are permitted to make partner brands part of their shows rather than distinct from them – an approach with which I had been familiar back in Canada. At Smooth, we were pleased to deliver successive deals with Foxy Bingo for the show, and I tried my best to honour the agreement and contribute in any way I could.

The Smooth Radio format, however, puzzled me somewhat. Although the brand name was Smooth, the station played the likes of Elvis and Roy Orbison, who have many excellent qualities, but whose signature music can rarely be defined as smooth. In the US, a smooth jazz format, for example, is truly that. In my view, Magic seemed to have identified more of the right territory with its warm delivery and music mix, and that approach seemed to me to be a more fashionable listen.

Smooth was then owned by the press group Guardian Media, and I often wondered why they did not take full advantage of their radio stations in promoting the press title. In time, Smooth was acquired by Global Radio, by then the owner of GCap, Heart and LBC, and moved to London. Global became the dominant player in UK commercial radio, and the familiar Leicester Square building became home to yet more radio brands.

In the radio business there are only two certainties: you will begin a run on a programme or with a station, and you will end it. And when your employer is taken over, the likelihood of the latter grows. After just a couple of years on-air, my end at Smooth Radio came suddenly. As I finished a show one day and packed up my headphones, the internal phone rang. Given it was the time of day when most bosses would usually have long since left the building, it was an ominous sign.

I was asked to be in the adjacent studio in five minutes. Global Radio programmer Dick Stone greeted me to deliver the news that I had just completed my final show on Smooth. I was assured it was nothing to do with me, the show or my audience figures – a sentence which always begs a question. When he suggested that I might have seen the decision coming, I assured him I had not. I was then escorted out the building. I felt sorry for Dick having to deliver the news, and as we walked to the door, I shook his hand and reassured him I appreciated he was simply doing his job. He was doing someone else's uncomfortable work for them.

It was six days before Christmas.

Leaving a radio station is always a tough experience. You care about what you do, you work hard, and you build a relationship with the audience, spending hours every day with them. A farewell is sad even at the best times, but when dismissed summarily, there is no chance to say goodbye. It is not about the money – most radio stations discharge their contractual obligations whether you are on-air or not – it is the feeling that you have walked out on your friends: the listeners.

Even in the crazy world of radio, I believe that most people are trustworthy when trusted. Had I been given a chance to host some final programmes, I would have behaved responsibly, just as Johnnie Walker did on his Radio 1 farewell show in 1976, even though he had left following a disagreement. Although there are some well-documented examples of angry presenters using their exit programmes on radio stations to platform about their treatment, it is relatively rare, and usually backfires long-term on the individual.

Listeners do respond sympathetically when the regular voice on the radio disappears and those comments are hugely welcome, although we all recognise that memories are short and the fans soon hopefully find some other presenter to their taste. The messages from other station staff are particularly reassuring, and, as I left Smooth I was touched to receive personal, supportive notes from leading people in the organisation.

More recently, I have enjoyed what I gather they call a portfolio career. It has taken me into welcome new areas such as through the doors of BBC local radio, a very different environment from commercial radio.

In Sussex and Surrey, I was on-air at the weekend so missed out a little on the weekday busy buzz of the station, but it was a pleasant surprise to bump into my old Capital colleague Graham Dene, who followed me on-air. The teams at the station were supportive, although I was struck how young many of them seemed to be, compared to the likely age of the audience. On some BBC local stations, I got the feeling that some of those on-air rather wished they were broadcasting somewhere else. Given their adaptive skills, however, it is perhaps not as bad as those themed compilation programmes on TV on a Saturday night where classic slices of Seventies and Eighties' TV are aired, accompanied by wry comment from 'talking heads' who were not even alive when the programmes were originally broadcast.

I appreciate the irony of those comments coming from this Kid, who was Radio Luxembourg's youngest presenter in 1968.

Remember the fast-moving TV ads for the famous *Now, That's What I Call Music* albums? Spawned from a Branson partnership between Virgin and EMI in 1983, the series succeeded the likes of the familiar K-Tel or Ronco LPs, delivering bundles of hits at pocket-money prices on the first-ever compilations. The first *Now* album I was charged with advertising breathlessly was *Now 8* in 1986, released in the days before the CD conquered all, and advertised as 'Thirty-two top chart hits on the ultimate double album and cassette', featuring hits from Duran Duran, Pet Shop Boys, Genesis, the Human League, Run-DMC and Kate Bush. How astonishing to realise that the series has now crashed through the *Now 100* mark. I enjoy my ongoing involvement with the *Now*

'70s TV channel, where I am one of the voices introducing clips of vintage hits.

Thanks to the boundless energy of former Luxembourg colleague Tony Prince and the support from my old Luxembourg colleague Golly Gallagher, I am also now part of the online station United DJs, to be found at www.uniteddj.com. Dubbed 'the station of the stars', UDJ involves many of the familiar DJ names from the days when radio was freer, and we could have more involvement in the music we chose to play. Most of my programmes are pre-recorded, piece by piece, with those links then slotted in between the music at the time the show is aired. It is good to learn the new skill of presenting a programme in a jigsaw fashion, although I do miss kicking back and relishing the experience of listening to great tracks in the context of what I say.

For many of the team at UDJ, it is a true passion project. For me, it is something to think about in the morning, and the value of that is inestimable. Positivity is so important in handling my medical condition, alongside eating well and exercising regularly. To a large extent, I decide when I wake whether I am to have a great day or not.

I accepted long ago that I now broadcast to smaller audiences than I used to, but amidst today's plethora of radio stations and unlimited streaming services, no presenter can command the heady heights that we did in the Seventies. In a sense, however, most of us in radio have never had audience size on our minds as we prepared our shows and threw open the fader. We just have a pride in doing the best we can for the listener who has chosen us.

27.

REFLECTIONS

At school, when I gazed up at the portrait of the jewelled Queen in my Vancouver classroom, I did not ever expect to be invited to dine with her family and a dozen others at a private reception at Frogmore House in Windsor Great Park.

As we drove up that day, Guðrún gestured through the passenger window to point out the Queen, wearing a headscarf, cantering alongside on her horse.

There are so many reasons to be thankful for the colourful life I have lived, which has afforded me the privilege of spending time with some of the greats in music whose legacy will never fade, and with radio colleagues whose friendship I have treasured.

I hope my happiness has never been at the expense of other people's. I am lucky to have made a life-long career simply doing what I enjoy. If anything, I proved a modest ordinary little lad could climb a mountain. A triumph for the little guy.

Although my accent ensures that I will always be perceived as Canadian, England has become home in my half a century here. Having said that, I adjusted quickly to the move from Canada and my mind easily wanders when I travel overseas. Italy is a place I love to visit and I feel I could live there, and I thoroughly enjoy the trips to see Guðrún's home country, Iceland. A stunning, quiet destination with dramatic weather conditions, it is invigorating to stroll around the harbour, seeing the massive freezer containers packed with the spoils of the sea.

Whilst I have witnessed talented people suffer from the excesses of the high life, with some paying the ultimate price, I would not wish to appear self-righteous in saying I have not been overly tempted. With alcohol, my body quickly tells me when a certain number of drinks is more than sufficient. Guðrún recalls that I only got 'pickled', as she calls it, once. It has been a few more times than that, but drunkenness is simply not something I am drawn to.

Of course, drug-taking has been in evidence in circles I have mixed in, but again it has simply not appealed. I am naturally hyperactive and do not feel the need for a stimulant; if I am to enjoy anything, I feel I need to be fully in control of my senses. I also have a deep dislike for those who have created an industry around the drugs which have brought the careers of so many talented people to a premature end.

During my Radio 1 days, Harry Nilsson called me, quite unexpectedly, asking me to lunch at a venue of my choice. Best known for his gut-wrenching vocal performance of 'Without You', I regarded him highly and he enjoyed an impressive following in his industry for the calibre of his song-writing. We agreed to meet at an Italian restaurant in Berkeley Square, and wandered to our seats downstairs. Looking up from the menu, he volunteered that I was probably wondering why I had been invited. I confessed I was. He began his lesson. 'You remind me of me. When I see you on *Top of the Pops*, you look like I used to. I don't now.' He went on to tell me how easy it was to become embroiled in a life of drink and drugs, and that he would hate for that to happen to me. Although not referred to in the conversation, Mama Cass had been found dead in Harry's flat in 1974. Harry himself would die aged just 52, in 1994. At our lunch, there was no further agenda whatsoever besides the friendly lecture on the evils of excess, and I was touched. I smiled, however, after dessert. 'Coffee?' asked the waitress. 'No,' replied Harry. 'But have you any Hine cognac?'

Harry was correct. Temptation of all sorts abounded. There was a stage when I was feted on arrival anywhere, and Guðrún found the attention I garnered difficult to believe. It was flattering to have women pay me interest but, as a married man, it was not my style to take advantage of the opportunities that a high profile presents for the most prosaic of reasons. I like my home; and even when working away, I always preferred to return there rather than stay overnight, wherever possible. Paul McCartney once told me that, at that time, he and Linda had never slept apart, preferring three hours in his own bed to nine hours somewhere else.

If wine, women and song are supposed to be the three key vices, I plead Guilty to the latter. Little compares with the feeling of being on-air, hosting a show you enjoy, playing music you feel passionate about and want to share with others, on a radio station with good colleagues where you feel valued. That is what has driven me.

Awards reflect some of those factors, not least when you are judged by your peers in broadcasting, or by listeners. I was delighted to win five Sony Radio Awards across my career, also being judged the New Spotlight DJ of the Year for 1972 and 1973. The *Melody Maker* DJ of the Year award in 1983 was a sweet victory, as the magazine had described me as sounding like the American cartoon character Huckleberry Hound when I made my on-air debut at Radio Luxembourg.

I won the *Variety* magazine award for Radio Personality title in 1980, the British Radio and Television Industry award for Best Radio Programme in 1986, and I received the Maple Leaf Award for Canadian Contribution to Broadcasting in 2002. In a straw poll for *Smash Hits*, I read I had been judged the 'Best DJ' by the unlikely trio of Rupert Everett, Terry Hall from the Specials and Siouxsie and the Banshees.

The recognition which touched me most was being added to the Radio Academy's Hall of Fame, where I feel almost uneasy sitting on the list amongst some of the UK greats from the earliest age of radio.

Another curious accolade was being declared a Freeman of the City of London in one of the oldest surviving traditional ceremonies, dating back to 1237. Technically, from the Middle Ages the Freedom was the right to trade in the Square Mile, but the title has been used in recent times simply to recognise special efforts.

The list of recipients includes the likes of Judi Dench, Nelson Mandela and Winston Churchill. In my humble case, the title was awarded for charity work. Like many of us, I have always tried to do my bit and had recently supported the work of the Bobby Moore Charity Fund for cancer research. Bobby, famously captain of England for the World Cup victory in 1966, died in 1993 aged just 51. We had bumped into each other numerous times over the years, particularly when he booked me for gigs at the pub he ran in East London.

The presentation ceremony was an affair deep in custom, with guests escorted by the Beadle in his top hat and frockcoat to the Chamberlain's Court at Guildhall. The Declaration was read before the Lord Mayor, Aldermen, Common Councilmen and invited guests, and the parchment on which the privilege is outlined in traditional calligraphy was handed over. That certificate remains on my wall to this day.

Friendships are formed for a reason, a season or a lifetime. Life in radio takes you from country to country, city to city, station to station. As you move on, you leave colleagues behind – but some remain lifelong friends. To this day, I still value Paul Burnett's company, and nothing will take away our shared perspective of life, founded on those heady days together in Luxembourg and at BBC Radio 1. He is a gifted storyteller, with more still to offer radio if the opportunity presented itself, and I relish meeting up with him.

It is also a privilege to spend time with Paul Gambaccini. When we travelled from place to place for events at Radio 1, I always seized the chance to grab a seat next to him on the coach. Such is his wry sense of humour, his memory, his music knowledge, his intelligence and his ability to put things in context, I felt flattered he wanted to spend time with me. His viewpoint is always worth listening to.

When Paul was under suspicion as part of the Yewtree investigations, I always felt confident that I knew him well enough to know that the allegations were lies, as was eventually conceded. It was such a relief to see him rightly exonerated and I cannot begin to imagine how one deals with that sort of situation. We met up for a few lunches during his twelve months of trauma, and he appeared to cope better on some occasions than others, sometimes down; but at other times more confident that right would prevail. Now the whole painful episode is over, it is right now that we think of Paul simply for his immense gifts and make full use of them. I was privileged recently to be invited to be his interviewer at a function at the Ivy Club in London.

Lynn Parsons lives down the road these days and has been hugely supportive. She is very much her own woman, yet a great listener. I really rate her on-air, with the lovely manner she has with listeners; never patronising, just an old-fashioned sincere approach. I know she is enjoying her excellent work at Magic, and BBC Radio 2 has missed out on her gifts.

Having moved abroad in my teens, leaving family and friends behind, the relationships here from the fields of both radio and music are particularly important to me.

It was a delight to be invited to Bill Wyman's 70th birthday party at Ronnie Scott's Jazz Club on Frith Street, and I enjoy the regular Radio Luxembourg and Radio 1 reunions where we gather over a drink or meal and re-tell stories we have shared a million times. The years are forgotten, the grey hairs ignored, and we just pick up where we left off.

I was privileged to be on-air at a pivotal stage in the journey of rock music and, just as I was making my name in radio, several key music figures were carving out their reputations in tandem. Having grown up in our respective colourful industries together, some of us feel a kinship and have remained in touch.

Although Wishbone Ash were to split into factions, as bands often do, lead singer and songwriter Martin Turner and I became friends, and his son Tom and my son Viktor and their respective families stay in touch to this day.

One warm Wishbone Ash memory is the gig to which I was invited by Martin at an atmospheric venue called Under The Bridge at Chelsea FC's home Stamford Bridge. Towards the end of their excellent set, he put his guitar down and paused to announce: 'Someone who means a lot to me is here tonight – and if you ever listened to Radio Luxembourg, you'll know him.' He then said my name and invited the crowd to stand and applaud. Such treasured moments are never forgotten.

Did I achieve everything I wanted in radio?

In 1987, during my time at Capital, MD Nigel Walmsley suggested I apply for the job as Head of Music, a post seen as next in line to programme director. Although I was thrilled by the faith being shown in me, and the encouragement from the wonderful Lynn Parsons, I did not feel I had the necessary credits for the job without any track record with senior management. I feel I am a better 'number two' than 'number one', a Peter Taylor rather than a Brian Clough. I am at my best helping someone else take an idea forward – and I love being on-air.

There have been uncertain times in my career, particularly in commercial radio. Although BBC contracts were short, the Corporation committed to those they had hired and there was an expectation that it would renew arrangements routinely, unless you erred seriously. I trusted the principled people I dealt with and felt I could look into their eyes and see truth.

I do not feel a career in music radio would now attract me in the way it did fifty years ago. With the growth in the number of stations and platforms, and the changes in the industry, I cannot imagine myself as a sixteen-year-old feeling the magic I felt all those years ago, nor having the confidence to insist I choose my own records. News media possibly would appeal to me now. Luck has played a huge part, and I recognise I was in the right place at the right time and lucky enough to be in the company of the right people, listening to the right advice. I strongly believe that where there is a will, there is a way, and when you know in your heart something can be achieved, it will be.

Whilst it was important for the UK's commercial radio stations to become more focussed on what they do in an ever-more competitive world, I fear I have witnessed some parts of the industry change inch-by-inch into one which risks becoming cold-blooded, with a prevailing atmosphere of fear, rather than fun. In recent years in the UK, presenter line-ups have been forever changing, with the team on-air never quite sure of their destiny, or even whether they were liked. There was little certainty that a contract would be renewed, even if eventually it was. Given listeners are not attracted to change, it is a puzzling approach.

Looking back, I wonder whether there were times in my radio life when I allowed myself to be bullied, just as I was at school until the day I was driven to retaliate. Maybe I should have spoken out more, and not simply accepted being cast as victim. Just as in football, I cannot agree that the best managers are bullies.

I still hope the best is yet to come for me in radio. I do miss the ethos of working regularly in a radio station building. Who would not wish to appear on BBC Radio 2? And now Radio 4 is opening its eyes to other accents apart from Home Counties, maybe they would consider mine? Having started out in classical music radio in Canada, it has been wonderful recently to be invited to guest on Radio 3's *Private Passions*.

In Luxembourg, radio dominated my days and nights, and I effectively lived on the job in the Villa Louvigny, now classified as a National Monument in that great city. Now, my pleasures come from my family, including my seven grandchildren, and in other areas of life.

Guðrún enjoys her work at the auctioneers Bonhams, and it plays to her gifts. Whenever we get in a lift in a building, by the time it reaches the desired floor, the occupants spill out laughing and Guðrún has made new friends. She has the knack of getting to know a wide range of people, and they instantly feel at ease with her. She is never forgotten.

Recently, we both attended an event at the House of Lords to mark an Icelandic festival. Usually, the mic is thrust at me in any event but, on this occasion, she volunteered to run the auction and took the opportunity to say a few words about her home country to the assembled throng of bow-tied luminaries. Without any preparation, she held the room, not least because of her familiar trait of scattering British idioms, delivered in her endearingly-accented English. Someone once said to me that she uses them so often, people begin to think she invented them.

My son Viktor shares my love of motor racing, driving the cars I would love to have done, clocking up speeds of 180mph at Rockingham Speedway in Corby. He did take Guðrún out for a whizz round the Brands Hatch circuit on one memorable occasion when her screams bounced off the walls of the nearby buildings.

He has loved cars since he rode go-karts as a kid, and soon started to take it seriously. At 16 he competed in Italy, and I still recall the thrill of hearing the roar of the engines and the excited announcer on the crackly public address speakers shouting 'Il Bambino' about Viktor as he motored into the lead. Pride in your children's achievements is a heady drug. Whilst I was willing him on trackside, Guðrún stood with her back to the track biting her nails with worry.

In 2007, Viktor raced in the British Formula Three International Championship with the Alan Docking Racing team, and in 2008 raced in the same series for Nexa Racing. I was told by Formula One executives that a lack of sponsorship was the only hurdle to his competing in truly top-flight racing, rather than any concerns about the calibre of his driving. Viktor is now settled in Hong Kong, doing well in the finance sector.

Although I would never be a driver myself, my own love for motorsport gave rise to the creation of Kid Jensen Racing. The days at the tracks I recall with huge fondness, arriving in the morning to the smell of sizzling bacon and coffees as we chatted with the mechanics and drivers before the excitement got underway. With two accomplished partners in Vincent Franceschini and Simon Barker, and equipment from Tyrrell Racing, we achieved some notable successes, becoming well-known in the Formula One paddock. Our finest hour came during the 1999 Grand Prix weekend at Silverstone, as Nicolas Minassian brought the car home, adorned with Jamiroquai's famous Medicine Man silhouette, to our maiden F3000 victory. I am proud to have had such an involvement in the sport, and treasure the memories.

Alexander also shares one of my passions, working as a news and sport broadcaster in radio, television and print since 2004. His break came at LBC in London, adding ESPN to his resume before basing himself in Korea from 2010. He is a gifted speaker, linguist and writer, and is doing well in both the media and communications in a vibrant and increasingly important part of the world. He has started his own family in Seoul, a city Guðrún and I have visited numerous times. For someone with my background, Korea is a wonderful blend of the familiar and the exotic.

My daughter Anna Lisa lives in the UK. She has a great brain and is a perennial student, now working for a PhD alongside the demands of looking after her three young children. She takes after me in terms of being quiet, something I appreciate people think radio presenters can never be.

Anna Lisa joined me years ago when I was filming a programme called *World Wise* from TVS for CITV, an excellent children's format which saw me sitting at a silver hydraulic desk which moved across a large map of the world. Contestants had to answer questions about countries to make progress to their destination, and victory. Anna Lisa was more fascinated by the programme being filmed in the studio afterwards, a wildlife show. Unlike me, she was more than happy to sink her hands in a container of tarantulas.

Despite the geographical distance between some of us, we all keep in touch and we are open, honest and close. We try to get together when we can, and manage the logistics for occasional wider family reunions with my siblings back in Canada – with a warm welcome guaranteed at Vancouver Airport before we adjourn for some of its legendary seafood at a coastline restaurant. My brother Lee is my best friend, eight years younger than me and a law enforcement officer there. Our younger sister Linda is retired, and loves her day walking around town and relishing the magnificent Vancouver skyline from her window.

I never saw much of my own dad after he left the family home in the Sixties. Being away in Luxembourg when my parents split originally, I was spared the most tumultuous period, and we lost contact. We children had been closer to my mother, who had been the larger influence growing up. She was fair, had decent values and a good sense of humour. I gather my dad met a new partner with family in England, who sent them British press cuttings featuring my radio and TV exploits. Those found their way back to my mother who, on one occasion, confided, 'Your father is proud of you.' It is odd that we shared the same career and yet did not stay close. He had dementia in later life and died a few years ago. At the end, I reflected, as one does, and wondered whether I should have been more gracious, putting my arm around him and finding closure... but it was not be.

Not every day is a good day as I live with my Parkinson's. It is easy to get depressed. I miss playing the sort of ball games we North Americans love, as I can no longer even throw one straight. I even find it difficult to do those fiddly necessary jobs which we take for granted, such as tying a necktie, putting on cufflinks or just fastening my trousers. It used to take twenty seconds to put on a shirt, now it can take twenty minutes. With Parkinson's you become reliant on other people, and I spare a thought for the people who cope alone.

Although the timbre of my voice may have just shifted a little, I am grateful that the tool of my trade remains intact.

On the tough days, I think of the uplifting recent words from a doctor at a specialist hospital in Epsom. Having measured my agility, stamina and strength, she suggested my performance was remarkable for someone who had lived with Parkinson's for the length of time I have. Advances in medicine are being made, and I gather we are tantalisingly close to finding a cure or, at least, managing the symptoms better than can be achieved currently. That gives me hope.

People now thoughtfully correct themselves when they address me as 'Kid' rather than David, but we are the same person. I shall always be Kid. Some fellow presenters shave off a year or two in their accounts of their life, but the name Kid is not about pretending to be young – it is who I am. I shall always be happy still to be Kid.

Over my career, several people I hold in high regard have suggested I should open-up more on-air about the real David Jensen. Who lives behind the voice? Although I have shown just a little more of myself in my programmes as my career has developed, I hope this book offers some insight into my life and how I have felt through a privileged journey.

Such is the nature of the radio business, the time in the sun for any radio presenter can be alarmingly brief. I have enjoyed the longest, warmest summer anyone could have wished for.

Of all the parts of my life I am grateful for, one is supreme. Without Guðrún by my side, caring, organising, pushing, scolding, giving me Icelandic tough love, and laughing, I doubt whether the rest would ever have come together.

MY MUSIC

There was a certain ceremony in the first playing of a newly-purchased vinyl album. Admiring the artwork, and reading every word of the cover notes. Then prising the record from its outer cover, and sliding the precious cargo gently from its white sleeve. After a dusting, holding it carefully, before placing the needle on the disc for the very first time and hearing that expectant crackle before the music kicks in.

Having disposed of my record collection when leaving the US, my own physical collection of product is now more limited. I did amass a collection of CDs on returning to the UK, including an autographed copy of the precious *Brothers in Arms* from Dire Straits which was amongst the first ever pop albums to be released on CD, with the medium confined to Classical works until that point. Mark Knopfler had been typically keen to embrace the best possible technology, and not only released it digitally on CD, but the recording sessions were digital too. Alas, my copy of that collectors' item was amongst a bundle that were stolen. My own music collections are clearly doomed.

I do now own a few CDs, but most of my music discovery these days is from the treasure trove of YouTube. Alongside the fresh releases, no matter how obscure the back catalogue track you seek, it is there.

But when it comes to great music, it matters not how you play it, provided the source is legitimate. What matters more is what happens inside your head when you hear it.

When I have friends over for dinner, I still get a kick from pulling out an album that my guests may not have yet heard before, and introducing it to them: 'Have a listen to this.' Is great music radio so different from that?

My favourite singles, in no particular order, include the following.

o   The Kinks: 'All Day And All Of The Night'. The Kinks have been one of my all-time favourite bands since childhood, and I have been lucky enough to see them live on a couple of occasions. Their riffs are almost primaeval, and I love the energy of this song.

o   The Buzzcocks: 'Ever Fallen In Love (With Someone You Shouldn't've)'. Lancashire's Pete Shelley was a frequent guest on my *Roundtable* on Radio 1, and this track means, to me, what 'Teenage Kicks' by the Undertones meant to John Peel.

o   The Beach Boys: 'Do It Again'. This track reminds me of my days on-air on CKOV back in Canada, when I had a hand in the music I played. Not the summer harmony side of the Beach Boys, but the more simplistic approach they did so well.

o   Thin Lizzy: 'Whiskey In The Jar'. Walking past a taxicab recently, I heard this song being played inside the vehicle. The driver looked up, pointed at me and gestured to his radio. We shared a smile. This is the song I was most associated with at Radio Luxembourg, having played it so often. Phil Lynott was a guest on the show frequently, although this is not a song he wrote; it dates back to the 17th century. It's the record which broke the band.

o   Barbara Lewis: 'Hello Stranger'. This has been recorded several times, but this is the original 1964 version, written by Barbara herself, as were all the songs on her debut LP. It's a great song about welcoming someone back to the fold when they have been away for some time, inspired by her early days on the circuit accompanying her musician father to familiar venues, when people called out fondly, 'Hello stranger' upon his return.

○ **Box Tops: 'The Letter'.** From Memphis, the Box Tops are often cited as being influential – and this 1967 track by that American band is era-defining, with an unusual construction. As every presenter knows, it is a conveniently short song, under two minutes in length, which made the Top Ten in the UK and reached Billboard's Number One position for four weeks.

○ **Eddie Cochran: 'Somethin' Else'.** Eddie was my real rock'n'roll hero. An experimental pioneer in the studio, even getting his producer to play a cardboard box with two rulers on 'Summertime Blues'. Sadly I never saw him live, but John Peel told me of his extraordinary performance. This song was covered brilliantly by the Sex Pistols – but Eddie's interpretation will always be best.

○ **Depeche Mode: 'Never Let Me Down Again'.** An adventurous song from a band which is underrated in the UK, but better recognised in the US. Depeche Mode deliver very appealing commercial songs, and were flag-bearers for electronica.

○ **Clifford T Ward: 'Home Thoughts From Abroad'.** This sad but utterly pictorial song is just immaculate with such a great lyric, which refers to his home county of Worcestershire. Hearing it during my months in the US made my eyes teary, thinking back to the country I now called home. Clifford came out to Luxembourg, and I picture him in the studio with long hair, softly spoken, playing his song 'Gaye' on his guitar. This ex-teacher never enjoyed the commercial success his songwriting warranted, although his work was loved by so many radio presenters including Terry Wogan, who cited this as his favourite song from the Queen's reign.

○ **Althea and Donna: 'Uptown Top Ranking'.** Althea Forrest and Donna Reid from Jamaica recorded this when they were just 17 and 18-years-old, and it was huge. I remember introducing them on *Top of the Pops*. Famously, the track was said to have been played on-air by John Peel – by accident.

○

MY FAVOURITE ALBUMS
Marvin Gaye: *What's Going On* (1971)
Miles Davis: *Kind of Blue* (1959)
Beach Boys: *Pet Sounds* (1966)
Van Morrison: *Astral Weeks* (1968)
Jimi Hendrix Experience: *Are You Experienced?* (1967)
Bruce Springsteen: *Born in the USA* (1984)
Beatles: *Revolver* (1966)
Aretha Franklin: *Lady Soul* (1968)
Bob Dylan: *Another side of...* (1964)
The Clash: *London Calling* (1979)
The Smiths: *Hatful of Hollow* (1984)
Elbow: *Seldom Seen Kid* (2008)
Hank Williams: *40 Greatest Hits* (1978)
Johnny Cash: *At Fulsom Prison* (1968)
Sting: *Live in Berlin* (2010)
Mark Knopfler: *Sailing to Philadelphia* (2000)
Ray Charles: *The Genius of Ray Charles* (1959)
Billy Bragg: *Mermaid Avenue* (1998)
Art Pepper: *Winter Moon* (1981)
Kate Bush: *Hounds of Love* (1985)
U2: *The Joshua Tree* (1987)
Peter Gabriel: *So* (1986)
Rolling Stones: *Exile On Main Street* (1972)
Led Zeppelin: *Led Zeppelin IV* (1971)
Joni Mitchell: *Court and Spark* (1974)

Frank Sinatra: *Strangers in the Night* (1966)
Nina Simone: *Baltimore* (1978)
Neil Young: *After the Gold Rush* (1970)
Santana: *Caravanserai* (1972)
Yes: *Close to the Edge* (1972)

INDEX

INDEX